SELECTED ISSUES IN GLOBAL HEALTH COMMUNICATIONS

Edited by **Muhiuddin Haider**
and **Heather Nicole Platter**

Selected Issues in Global Health Communications
http://dx.doi.org/10.5772/intechopen.72462
Edited by Muhiuddin Haider and Heather Nicole Platter
Assistant to the Editor(s): Bridget L. Higginbotham

Contributors

Muhiuddin Haider, Anton Schneider, Emily Haas, Patrick Yorio, Jiyoung An, Jinkyung Paik, Paulo Meira, Ilana Trombka, Daniele Mendes, Mohsen Shams

Notice

Statements and opinions expressed in the chapters are these of the individual contributors and not necessarily those of the editors or publisher. No responsibility is accepted for the accuracy of information contained in the published chapters. The publisher assumes no responsibility for any damage or injury to persons or property arising out of the use of any materials, instructions, methods or ideas contained in the book.

First published in London, United Kingdom, 2018 by IntechOpen
IntechOpen is the global imprint of INTECHOPEN LIMITED, registered in England and Wales, registration number: 11086078, The Shard, 25th floor, 32 London Bridge Street
London, SE19SG – United Kingdom
Printed in Croatia

British Library Cataloguing-in-Publication Data
A catalogue record for this book is available from the British Library

Additional hard copies can be obtained from orders@intechopen.com

Selected Issues in Global Health Communications, Edited by Muhiuddin Haider and Heather Nicole Platter
p. cm.
Print ISBN 978-1-78923-789-4
Online ISBN 978-1-78923-790-0

We are IntechOpen,
the world's leading publisher of
Open Access books
Built by scientists, for scientists

3,700+
Open access books available

116,000+
International authors and editors

119M+
Downloads

Our authors are among the

151
Countries delivered to

Top 1%
most cited scientists

12.2%
Contributors from top 500 universities

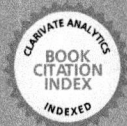

Interested in publishing with us?
Contact book.department@intechopen.com

Numbers displayed above are based on latest data collected.
For more information visit www.intechopen.com

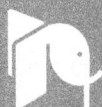

Meet the editors

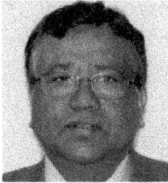

Muhiuddin Haider, PhD, is Clinical Professor in Global Health at the University of Maryland School of Public Health's Institute for Applied Environmental Health. Since 2009, he has been teaching undergraduate courses under the Public Health Science and Global Health Scholars Programs, while also teaching graduate-level courses in the Global Health Certificate Program offered through the University of Maryland School of Public Health. In addition to teaching, Dr. Haider is currently a coinvestigator in Project HEAL: Health through Early Awareness and Learning, an intervention to increase cancer screening in African American faith-based communities in Prince Georges County, Maryland. He is also the Principal Investigator on a study to assess the US Public Health Service Commissioned Corps Officers' value to public health.

Dr. Haider is a highly skilled public health professional who has managed and led diverse public health projects and research studies in more than a dozen countries worldwide over the past 30 years on behalf of several international agencies and universities. He has assisted multisector initiatives to advance the delivery of quality healthcare services in the areas of avian influenza, HIV/AIDS, TB, RH/FP, and malaria, and has developed expertise in the areas of health communication, health promotion, health education, and social marketing. His research into strategies of behavior change, application of social marketing tools, and communications capacity building has led to several acclaimed publications.

He has led major public health projects in several countries in Africa and Asia, for which he utilized technical skills to stimulate innovative and culturally sensitive approaches grounded in organizational and technical soundness. His recent research and programmatic work has focused on avian and pandemic influenza, for which he has contributed to creating and adapting IEC, BCC, and IPC training materials to establish and implement best practices within public healthcare systems and promote public/private partnerships.

Dr. Haider has worked collaboratively on numerous occasions with counterparts in the veterinary and agriculture sectors and has advanced the "One World, One Health" framework through curriculum development, targeted coursework for public health students, and the development of a concept paper endorsed by the DOD Veterinary Service Activity, Princeton University-based One Health Initiative Advocacy Group, Agricultural Research Service, DOA, and WHO. Dr. Haider has developed and conducted training sessions for media/health reporting, with special focus on AI through DOS/VOA and IBB. Recently, Dr. Haider was awarded a Fulbright Scholar Grant to assist the Ecuadorian Nutritional Program, Universidad De Saint Francisco in Quito.

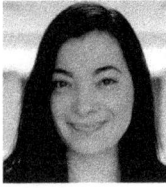

Heather Nicole Platter is a doctoral candidate in Behavioral and Community Health in the School of Public Health at the University of Maryland. She completed her Bachelor and Master of Science from the University of Florida. Heather worked in Peru for many years to improve child health in rural communities by implementing community health worker programs. Additionally, she managed a Peruvian organization to improve access to post-secondary education for youths with disabilities. She is currently a research fellow at the Horowitz Center for Health Literacy. Her research interests include health communication, health literacy, tobacco control and cancer prevention, health behavior, and global health. Her dissertation is a grounded theory study exploring health literacy barriers to screening for lung cancer.

Contents

Preface

Introduction

This book was written to give scholars an opportunity to examine selected issues in health communication. There are many challenges in health communication, such as the shortage of evaluations on social marketing interventions, the need for a framework to easily apply social marketing practices to campaigns, and the difficulty of applying theory to improve communication. To address these challenges, the following four chapters, including an introductory chapter, introduce several health communication topics, including social marketing, the application of theory, and message design to promote social communication. Readers can expect concise topic overviews with clear steps and examples of how to apply the methods discussed in each chapter.

Chapter Summaries

Chapter 1: Introduction: Focused on Issues and Challenges in Global Health Communication

Over the years, social and behavior change (SBC) has accumulated a robust body of compelling evidence, consisting of both scientific research and documented success stories that demonstrate how the tools and approaches of SBC have effectively influenced behavior change in almost every area of public health, as well as related sectors. The many adoptions of creative products and services that have been developed within the field make it easy for policy makers and program implementers to see that art and creativity play an important role in SBC.

Chapter 2: Using Sensemaking Theory to Improve Risk Management and Risk Communication: What Can We Learn?

This chapter introduces the topics of risk management and communication, as well as a model on the identification and mitigation of hazards using sensemaking theory to improve interpersonal communications and subsequent decision making. For risk communication to facilitate sensemaking, the authors advise distinctiveness, consistency, and consensus. Through the sensemaking process, individuals are expected to change behavior by taking responsibility and perceiving risks to identify and prevent accidents. In addition to introducing the four components of sensemaking, this chapter reviews the five stages of the traditional risk management cycle.

Chapter 3: Healthcare Message Design Toward Social Communication: Convergence Based on Philosophical and Theoretical Perspectives

This chapter presents the emerging concept Healthcare Message Design (HMD), which entails the use of interdisciplinary science to develop effective communication mechanisms with the goal of improving health outcomes and facilitating the healing process. The authors illustrate HMD using a hybrid model made up of three phases: theoretical, fieldwork, and analytical. This chapter expands on the theoretical phase of the model and defines the four attributes of HDM, which include concepts (healthcare, design, and communication), an interdisciplinary approach, meanings and measurements, and working conditions.

Chapter 4: Social Marketing for Health: Theoretical and Conceptual Considerations

This chapter begins by introducing a set of benchmark criteria for social marketing interventions, which will allow users to utilize key concepts of social marketing to increase the impact of an intervention. Additionally, this chapter presents the Social Marketing Assessment and Response Tool (SMART), a social marketing planning model that encompasses seven phases to successfully plan a social marketing intervention. Further, this chapter explores the successful implementation of social marketing to (1) reduce risky driving behaviors among taxi drivers, (2) increase the use of helmets and safety masks among construction workers, (3) promote mammograms to women over 35, and (4) promote normal vaginal delivery among pregnant mothers considering a cesarean section.

Chapter 5: Social Marketing and Health Communication: A Case Study at the Brazilian Federal Senate

This chapter provides an overview of social marketing and internal marketing as powerful tools that institutions can use to achieve effective health communication. The utility of these marketing tools is highlighted with a case study on Pink October, the 2017 Brazilian Federal Senate month-long campaign for breast cancer. The campaign was brought together by an interdepartmental and interinstitutional partnership and utilizes social marketing and internal marketing concepts to achieve social change. Since challenges remain regarding the assessment of effective social marketing programs, the authors evaluate the campaign through the use of focused interviews, analysis of media articles, and a literature review. The results of the evaluation include the strengths of the campaign as well as the challenges and concerns that will need to be improved upon in future years.

Closing

The chapters in this book challenge the approach and deepen the understanding of health communication under a holistic model where health systems and public health are connected. The case studies used in the chapters provide an in-depth analysis of the complexities that exist in the health sector enterprise and the balance between health products, human behavior change, and social benefits.

Both theoretical and methodological analyses represent an enormous step forward in commercializing social awareness and social marketing fully in the field of health communication implementation. Insights into the practice of social cognition theory are invaluable for any serious reader of behavioral economics in this contemporary society.

The centrality of addressing the public health trust and influences of marketing interests in campaign messages make this book an essential contribution to the capacity building of public health and health communication. Efforts in capacity building should address: (1) optimizing biomedical approaches, (2) reducing risk behaviors, (3) modifying unhealthy behaviors, and (4) shifting norms that have the potential to influence individual and collective behavior in the long term. Given the numerous challenges in health communication, we hope these chapters are able to assist scholars in addressing health communication challenges at the theoretical, methodological, and best practice levels.

For further reading

Haider, Muhiuddin (2005). Global Public Health Communication, Jones and Bartlett Publishers, Boston

Obregon, Rafael and Waisbord, Silvio (2012). The Handbook of Global Health Communication, Wiley-Blackwell , Meldon

Rogers, Everett M. (2003). Diffusion of Innovations (Fifth Edition), Free Press, New York

Zimmerman, Rick S., DiClemente, Ralph J., Andrus, Jon K., and Hosein, Everold N. (2016). Society for Public Health Education, Jossey-Bass, San Francisco

The Communication Initiative: www.comminit.org

The Health Compass: www.thehealthcompass.org

Muhiuddin Haider
Clinical Professor in Global Health
University of Maryland
College Park, MD, USA

Heather Nicole Platter
School of Public Health
University of Maryland
College Park, MD, USA

Bridget L. Higginbotham
Assistant to the Editor
University of Maryland
College Park, MD, USA

Introduction

Introductory Chapter: Global Health Communication - Focused Issues and Challenges

Anton Schneider and Muhiuddin Haider

Additional information is available at the end of the chapter

http://dx.doi.org/10.5772/intechopen.80674

1. Introduction

The current art and science of social and behavior change (SBC) has benefited from the many lessons learned and documented over the years from a wide variety of disciplines and approaches—including anthropology, psychology, marketing, communication research, social marketing, and more recently behavioral economics and human-centered design. Over the years, SBC has accumulated a robust body of compelling evidence, consisting of both scientific research, and documented success stories that demonstrate how the tools and approaches of SBC have effectively influenced behavior change in almost every area of public health, as well as related sectors. The many creative products and events that have been developed within the field make it easy for us to see that art and creativity play an important role in SBC. However, the science behind SBC is less visible but has, arguably, been even more important to the field's success.

In what might be the birth of social marketing 1951, Weibe famously asked the question "Why can't we sell brotherhood the way we sell Coca Cola?" [1, 2]. As in Weibe's famous paper, SBC has, from its earliest days, sought to identify, document, and implement the most effective means of influencing individual and community adoption of improved practices, whether these were technological or behavioral innovations, to improve health status. Central to his inquiry was the search for an approach that could provide results at scale for good value. And these efforts have been successful. Working in concert with the introduction of innovations from the biomedical field, SBC has contributed to significant reductions in mortality and increases in lifespan in every area of the globe. In recent years, we have seen an accelerated effort to document the evidence for SBC's effectiveness [3]. For example, in 2013, the United States Agency for International Development (USAID), in collaboration with the UNICEF, hosted the *Evidence Summit on Enhancing Child Survival and Development in Lower- and*

Middle-Income Countries by Achieving Population-Level Behavior Change in Washington, DC. The goal of the summit was to determine which evidence-based interventions and strategies support a sustainable shift in health-related behaviors in populations in lower- and middle-income countries to reduce under-5 morbidity and mortality. The results—documented in a special supplement to the Journal of Health Communication—clearly showed the tremendous successes in behavior change programs while carving a path forward to identify the most significant challenges and gaps for further exploration and research [4].

1.1. Adoption of products and services

It has long been recognized that simply having great products or services was insufficient, if people were unwilling to use them. This is the classic problem of "building a better mousetrap." The product can only be successful if people recognize the problem, are aware of the solution, find the solution beneficial, know where to obtain the product, find the outlets to be convenient, have the means and willingness to pay, and the list goes on. The public health equivalent is the myriad services and products that have been proven to improve health if only they are adopted. For example, in the earliest years of international development, the USAID and other donors provided family planning and child health technologies, such as contraceptives, oral rehydration solution, and vaccines, to countries with very high rates of child and maternal mortality. They quickly realized that, in order for these new technologies to be successful, they would need to be paired with behavioral interventions to promote adoption, proper use, and adherence. Later, similar strategies were used to increase demand for services, such as skilled delivery and antenatal care visits among pregnant women. It was the behavioral response—adoption of the technological innovation—no less than the innovation itself, that proved crucial to achieve the health outcome. "Better" technologies, like better mousetraps, cannot be effective when communities do not use them or do not use them correctly. Today, we have even more amazing technologies, such as ARVs, rapid diagnostic tests for malaria, PrEP for prevention of HIV, and GeneXpert machines that can distinguish drug-sensitive from drug-resistant TB, with new innovations appearing every day. Optimizing the life-saving potential of these technologies means using the full suite of available behavior change tools and approaches to connect these new technologies with the audience segments that can most benefit from their adoption and use. It also requires effective partnerships and close coordination to ensure that behavioral interventions are well synchronized and coordinated with supply-side sectors such as R&D, service delivery, product distribution, and information systems.

1.2. Prioritize customer experience

Numerous public health strategies, for example, WHO's End TB Strategy, remind us to develop "patient-centered" approaches [5]. Nevertheless, public sector approaches, especially those in resource-poor settings, often struggle with issues of adequate supplies, staffing, and properly functioning equipment and supplies. Historically, public health has tended to prioritize biomedical over behavioral interventions and adherence to clinical protocols over consumer experience. After all, patients tend to be poor judges of the real quality of clinical care. As every marketer and retailer knows, consumers tend to prioritize subjective qualities such as convenience, friendliness, and appearance. Marketers naturally understand that it is important to be attentive to consumer experience and generally do this better than the public sector. Despite the advantages, this also has its drawbacks, for example, patients can be attracted to substandard care in the private sector, both formal and informal, avoiding more effective alternatives available in a public system fraught with long lines, limited hours, staffing problems, and poor customer service. However, increasingly, public health practitioners realize that, in order to achieve the ambitious health goals that have been set, such as SDG 2030 Goal 3, new tools will be needed and the consumer perspective will need to be featured more prominently [6]. In recent years, in order to bridge this gap, new tools, such as human-centered design (HCD) and nudging, are being adapted from the commercial sector and quickly taken up. Such approaches—that place the customers' experience at the center of their strategy—are being increasingly adopted and evaluated, in order to increase uptake of priority practices, reduce the gap between clinical and consumer perceptions of quality, and lead to better health outcomes [7, 8].

1.3. Identify behavioral bottlenecks

There are a class of diseases, often termed as "lifestyle diseases," which include atherosclerosis, heart disease, stroke, obesity, and type 2 diabetes and diseases associated with smoking, alcohol, and drug abuse. Most people are well aware that lifestyle changes—such as regular physical exercise combined with a healthy diet—can help reduce the risk of such serious diseases and lead to a longer better quality life, yet they do not act on what they know so well. Research has shown that these diseases can often be prevented by "simple" modifications in lifestyle behaviors such as eating a healthy diet, regular exercise, avoiding tobacco, and getting proper sleep. This begs the often asked question "why don't people do what is good for them," or why do not people act (more) rationally? If people acted rationally, we would not see these diseases at the levels we do. Nevertheless, changing such lifestyle behaviors has proven challenging, involving the full spectrum of SBC approaches to affect all of the factors that can influence decision-making. These include (1) internal factors such as knowledge, attitudes, and beliefs; (2) social factors such as social norms, traditional practices, and the influence of important others; and (3) structural factors such as policies, regulations, and changes in the physical environment that determine access, convenience, and availability.

"Why won't people do what is best for them?" is a question that has challenged the field of behavior change since its origins and has led us to go beyond addressing individual factors (such as awareness, knowledge, and beliefs) to address the social and structural factors that can have such a powerful influence on individual behaviors. This fight has recently been joined by behavioral economists (BE) who have developed a new field that bridges economics and behavioral sciences to provide a fresh perspective on the seemingly irrational human decision-making and behavior. The field of behavior change has expanded and benefited significantly from the emergence and broad acceptance of this new field and the fresh perspective and tools it provides. Brought into the public spotlight in the past several years, through several best-selling books, as well as numerous podcasts, TED talks, and other popular media, behavioral economics has been able to shed new light on human behavior and what shapes behavioral choice. The BE practitioners have been rewarded not only with popular acceptance but have also been awarded the Nobel Prize in economics three times between 1992 and 2017. BE's contributions to SBC are relatively recent, so another of our key challenges will be to fully document how significant its contributions can be.

1.4. Negotiate behavior change

For the past 60 years or more, social causes and public health programs have adopted all manners of media to inform and persuade, often to good effect, especially when media channels were combined and paired with interpersonal means of community engagement. Disease outbreaks in recent years have offered an opportunity to examine the role that various forms of communication play as communities and outside experts work and struggle to negotiate local solutions. The West African Ebola outbreak 2014–2015 clearly showed that media was able to quickly and broadly convey information about the risk to audiences near and far. However, suspicion and rumors could also spread quickly through social media and social networks and just as quickly lead to detrimental results. We also saw that medical solutions could be stalled or ineffective without community dialog and effective, negotiated community engagement [9]. Disease outbreaks such as Ebola have clearly shown that communities need to be engaged from the outset, and, if their concerns are ignored, they can mobilize to thwart the efforts of public health workers. In outbreak situations, decisions must be made quickly, so it is not uncommon to find a small village besieged by technical experts from the outside—whether from the district, the capital, or other countries. It should not be surprising that communities that have become accustomed to receiving few services from the outside may be suspicious of the sudden attention, and it is not unusual for rumors to spring up questioning the motives of the outsiders. "Community engagement" has become the broadly accepted term to describe the strategy for creating dialog with communities to gain or regain their trust and cooperation in the face of an outbreak or other unusual health event. An important aspect of community engagement is the recognition that behaviors are not determined solely by individuals. The "social" in social and behavior change is important because individual choice has its limits and behaviors often involve social norms, traditions, and taboos. In order to successfully influence individuals to make better choices, we need to engage social networks effectively, for example, by building on the important roles played by respected leaders in the community and elders within the family [10]. For example, during the Ebola crisis, traditional burial practices and customs were found to be a major conduit of disease transmission. However, the solution was not to end traditional practices. Community leaders and technical experts worked with experts in SBC, including anthropologists, to find out ways to accommodate traditional beliefs and practices in behaviors that were also effective in stopping transmission.

2. Looking forward

The field of SBC has come so far from its origins in the middle of the last century. Over the years, it has built a strong evidence base, demonstrating the link between health outcomes and key behaviors. Moreover, through science and practice we now have a broad and robust set of tools and approaches available to identify and address the individual, social, and structural factors that influence behaviors. We have gone from simple awareness-raising campaigns to the use of scientific methods to build evidence-based approaches. In order to achieve the ambitious 2030 SDG health goals, however, SBC will need to provide support to the technological innovations that will be necessary and can only realize their potential if they are adopted and put to use. And technological breakthroughs are not limited to the medical field. We should expect that the important media technologies that connect our communities will also continue to evolve. Even potential disruptive policy solutions, such as Universal Health Care (UHC), will need to draw on SBC approaches to influence policymakers; target and monitor uptake among key audiences, such as lower-income or marginalized audience segments; and educate providers.

To meet these challenges, we'll need to continue to develop and draw on behavioral science, have an open mind, be open to new learning, and continue to add to the evidence base of what works and what does not. We will need to work and coordinate ever more effectively across multiple sectors and across ever more partners, defining roles and responsibilities so as to optimize the contributions of our various contributing partners—host country governments, multilateral agencies, international and local implementing partners, community-based groups, NGOs, donors, media, research agencies, and local communities themselves. We'll need the field to continue to develop tools and advocate for approaches that bring the consumer experience to the central focus of strategic design, implementation, and research. After all, SBC must continue to prioritize the voluntary nature of behaviors and the importance of incorporating community sensibilities, traditions, and preferences. We need to strive to ensure that respect for our key audiences, especially the poorest and most marginalized, is brought to the front and center of considerations regarding planning and implementation. In that spirit, practitioners should strive to elevate the experience of the humble villager and represent their perspective at the decision-making table with more powerful policymakers and technical experts where strategies are developed and implementation plans are drawn up. As behavior change planners, researchers, and practitioners, we should strive to sharpen our instruments to identify and address the factors that will reduce the barriers to behavior change for our beneficiaries so as to make voluntary behavior change as positive experience as possible. And lastly, we will need to keep an eye on the needs of policymakers and funders because the decision to fund behavior change approaches ultimately rests on our ability to provide solid evidence that SBC can deliver health outcomes at scale for a good value.

Author details

Anton Schneider[1]* and Muhiuddin Haider[2]

*Address all correspondence to: aschneider@usaid.gov

1 USAID, Bureau of Global Health, Office of Infectious Disease, GHSI-III—CAMRIS International, Inc., Washington, DC, USA

2 Global Health, University of Maryland, College Park, MD, USA

References

[1] Kotler P, Zaltman G. Social marketing: An approach to planned social change. Journal of Marketing. 1971;**35**(3):3-12

[2] Wiebe GD. Merchandising commodities and citizenship on television. Public Opinion Quarterly. 1951;**15**(4):679-691. DOI: 10.1086/266353

[3] Waisbord S. Where do we go next? Behavioral and social change for child survival. Journal of Health Communication. 2014;**19**(suppl 1):216-222. DOI: 10.1080/10810730.2014.933288

[4] Fox E, Obregon R. Population-level behavior change to enhance child survival and development in low- and middle-income countries. Journal of Health Communication: International Perspectives. 2014;**19**(suppl 1):3-9. DOI: 10.1080/10810730.2014.934937

[5] World Health Organization. The End TB Strategy [Internet]. 2018. Available from: http://www.who.int/tb/post2015_TBstrategy.pdf?ua=1 [Accessed: July 31, 2018]

[6] Sustainable Development Knowledge Platform [Internet]. 2017. Available from: https://sustainabledevelopment.un.org/sdg3 [Accessed: July 31, 2018]

[7] Brown T, Wyatt J. Design thinking for social innovation. Stanford Social Innovation Review. Winter. 2010

[8] Thaler RH, Sunstein CR. Nudge: Improving Decisions about Health, Wealth, and Happiness. 1st ed. Penguin Books; 24 February 2009. p. 320. ISBN-13: 978-0143115267

[9] Storey JD, Chitnis K, Obregon R, Garrison K. Community engagement and the communication response to Ebola. Journal of Health Communication. 2017;**22**(suppl 1):2-4. DOI: 10.1080/10810730.2017.1283200

[10] Berg RC, Denison E. A tradition in transition: Factors perpetuating and hindering the continuance of female genital mutilation/cutting (FGM/C) summarized in a systematic review. Health Care for Women International. 2013;**34**(10):837-859

Theory and Concepts

Using Sensemaking Theory to Improve Risk Management and Risk Communication: What Can We Learn?

Emily J. Haas and Patrick L. Yorio

Additional information is available at the end of the chapter

http://dx.doi.org/10.5772/intechopen.75725

Abstract

Risks and communication surrounding risks must be interpreted and responded to by employees in a way that honors the organization's health and safety (H&S) goals. This chapter integrates sensemaking theory and organizational risk management processes. In doing so, information is gleaned about gaps in risk communication messaging and dissemination. This proposed model has the potential to enhance the organizational and communication processes necessary to support the cognitive, motivation, and social coordination components in risk communication messaging that underlie H&S decision making.

Keywords: behavior change, decision making, health and safety management systems, risk communication, risk management, sensemaking

1. Introduction to risk management and communication

Health, safety, and risk management systems are designed to establish and achieve occupational goals, serving as primary mechanisms to control risks in the workplace [1, 2]. Their effectiveness in preventing loss and harm, however, depends upon the execution of behaviors necessitated by this overarching system. Despite the continued emphasis on the importance of organized action in risk management (RM) activities throughout the plan-do-check-act cycle, research suggests that implementation efforts often fail due to misinterpretation [1, 3, 4]. Although much effort has been dedicated to the behavioral aspects of RM primarily in the form of leadership/communication theories [5–10], organizational climate theories [8, 11–13], and knowledge/motivation theories [14–16], as a discipline we lack a framework that provides relevant information around RM practices including workplace risk identification, perception, and mitigation. As a result, cognitive, motivational, and social coordinative components in the workplace cease to evolve [17]. Mainly, because all employees are responsible for executing strategic health and safety (H&S) goals, it is challenging to track, troubleshoot, and control the entire system across managers, workers, shifts, job processes, and changing hazards [18–21]. Also, little theoretical work has been postulated to help understand the process by which risk practices are behaviorally executed throughout a continuous risk cycle [20, 22, 23].

The purpose of this chapter is to build upon an existing framework—sensemaking theory—to enhance the risk communication surrounding cognitive and motivational fundamentals of H&S behavior. This chapter makes one of the first attempts to formally integrate sensemaking theory with the cyclical RM process and thereby more formally explains the theoretical processes that link organizational health and safety management systems theory with behavior-based systems theory. We intentionally design the argument and theoretical application to be generalizable across high-risk occupations, and as a result, avoid contextualizing this framework using industry-specific examples. Thus, the goal of this chapter is to provide a model that can be adapted to integrate sensemaking and the accompanying organizational and communicative components needed to facilitate risk management within any high-risk organization to identify and mitigate hazards.

2. Traditional risk management cycle

Five stages are often included in a continuous RM cycle [24–26]. First, *risk identification* consists of identifying a hazard or acknowledging a risk [27]. Common examples include accident records, root cause analysis, hazard inspections, and workplace audits [28, 29]. *Risk assessment* is the process of determining if the hazard poses an unacceptable risk that could result in an incident and therefore, needs to be reduced to prevent an incident [1, 27]. *Risk mitigation* incorporates the "plan" and "do" of the H&S management cycle via the development and implementation of previously developed RM strategies (e.g., machine guarding, work flow, building design, proper/adequate equipment and tools, personal protective equipment) and includes all those involved in the risk [28–30]. A *risk response* entails any type of follow-up effort to mitigate the hazard such as elimination, reporting/placing a work order, or changing a work task or behavior to minimize the threat [1]. Finally, *risk monitoring* encompasses continued observation and awareness of the hazard [27]. Organizations select various sets of distinct practices aligned with each phase of the RM cycle [28]. Risk management practices include any action that can help prevent incidents, as well as enhance workplace perceptions and performance [26, 31].

2.1. The role of communication in managing risks

Risk communication is the "process of exchanging information among interested parties about the nature, magnitude, significance, or control of a risk" ([32], p. 359). This communication can entail a formal or informal estimate of whether something poses a high or low threat to personal safety and based on that perceived threat, how to respond [33]. Risks are best managed through consistent dialog between employees and managers [34, 35], and engaging employees in ongoing risk response and monitoring in order to build knowledge, awareness, and motivation of workers [36]. Communication is often noted as a basic component of RM, but several barriers exist that hinder risk communication between two entities within an organization.

2.2. Barriers that inhibit communication throughout the risk management cycle

Several barriers exist that hinder communicating about and executing risk practices to prevent incidents. One barrier is the varying levels of risk perception that individuals have and the potential for them to misjudge the potential severity of those hazards [37]. Reason [38] argues that "the inability of individuals being able to recognize and respect the full extent of operational hazards can lead to the creation of more and longer-lasting holes in the defensive layers" (p. 82). For example, previous research has pointed toward optimistic bias and overconfidence as a challenge in identifying and preventing incidents on site [39, 40]. Specifically, individuals in both occupational and recreational settings commonly discuss a low perceived likelihood that something bad will happen to them as a result of a hazard or risk in their space [41].

Another barrier is that everyone has responsibility throughout the RM cycle and, because an individual's or group's practices may be aligned with one phase of RM, it can be difficult for each person to understand how their role and decisions fit into the process. If such compartmentalization occurs, it is more likely that individuals cognitively interpret hazards and risks in a vacuum. For each individual to be clear about what actions are acceptable and unacceptable in preventing incidents [42], risk communication must be understood and responded to appropriately at all levels within an organization [43].

Last, even if individuals possess a sense of personal responsibility to mitigate risks and feel comfortable expressing concerns, the communication they receive about such risks must be perceived as important to respond efficiently and safely [44]. Without shared cognition and communication about these experiences, individuals are more likely to only observe bits and pieces of risk management with no reference as to how it "works" and fits into a more proactive process.

3. Incorporating sensemaking into risk management

Sensemaking has been applied as a communication tool and organizing framework to examine threats, risks, and hazards in the context of the healthcare industry [45–47], nuclear power plants [48], organizational crises and disaster response [49, 50], and gaps in organizational leadership [51]. Retrospective root cause analyses have also been framed to facilitate sensemaking within organizations in regard to RM activities [52]. Sensemaking is a process that can improve interpersonal communication when people must make decisions during extreme events and has been used to mitigate organizational crises [53]. To date, sensemaking has yet to be theoretically integrated into the RM cycle and remains absent in the literature that discusses dynamic workplace contexts [45, 53].

3.1. Overview of the sensemaking process

Because sensemaking can help engage workers in organizational RM, we focus on the process of sensemaking among receivers of messages to better understand how to communicate about risks and motivate participation in risk mitigation activities. Below, we debrief the four-step sensemaking process (i.e., *ecological change, enactment, selection,* and *retention*) (**Figure 1**).

First, to initiate sensemaking an event has to occur (*ecological change*) that is noticed by an individual, group, or organization. Examples include acknowledging the presence of the prescribed practices included within an organization's H&S goals, seeing a new workplace hazard or risk, or a co-worker/personal work-related injury. *Enactment* occurs when organizational leaders or workers choose to pay attention to the event [54]. After the event is noticed (*enactment*), the members of the organization must make sense of it and then do something about it (*selection*). At the worker level, *selection* entails choosing the appropriate behavioral response in accordance with the perceived meaning behind the H&S practices within the workplace. From a leadership level, *selection* entails deciding on the proper policy choice when responding to a previously unforeseen risk.

If these implemented responses and policy solutions are effective in reducing equivocality, they will likely be retained for subsequent sensemaking and become engrained into an organization's reaction to a situation [54]. Therefore, *selection* has important implications for long-term decisions and actions, as these decisions are often used to prevent future incidents or avoid injuries [55]. Eventually, *retention* occurs when ways of making decisions, handling workplace hazards, or preventing risky situations become part of an organization's policies, procedures, routines, and methods of organizing [56].

3.2. Risk recognition initiating ecological change

Cognitive recognition that a hazard exists is necessary before sensemaking begins. In the context of occupational health and safety it is the risk intertwined with job and task execution that must be recognized. This recognition is the beginning of a conscious decision to act upon what has been noticed. In the context of occupational H&S, however, because hazards inherent to work processes are likely to be encountered daily, both managers and workers can become used to "seeing" these hazards and in some ways, complacent or unaware of their presence [45]. Slip, trip, and fall hazards at occupational worksites is a common example.

In response, communication from leadership, situated in the middle of the integrated model (**Figure 2**), plays an important role in encouraging situational awareness of ecological changes

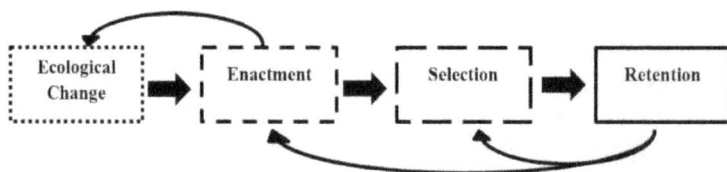

Figure 1. Organizational sensemaking process (Weick, 1999).

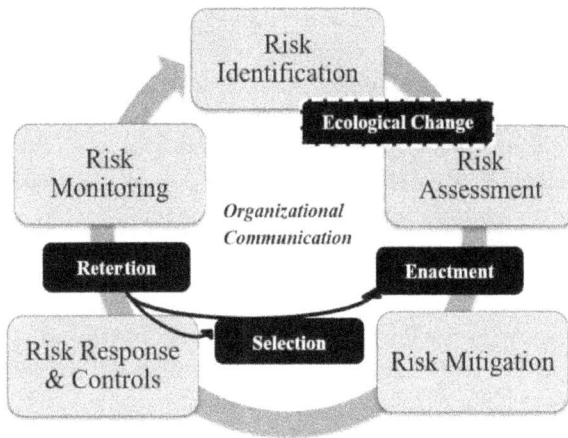

Figure 2. Sensemaking within the risk management cycle.

in the workplace—including the propensity to notice and the motivation to respond to potential hazards and present risks. From a management perspective, proactive hazard and risk identification activities are integral to the HSMS (e.g., job hazard analyses, health and safety audits, system safety studies, etc.). Workers must also be vigilant and seek out unanticipated hazards and risks that have passed through risk control activities unchecked. Tools such as pre-task job task briefings, worker self-checking, and stop-think-act-review activities are examples of practices often incorporated within behavior-based management systems that empower and engage workers in the first of the four step sensemaking process as well as planning within their RM processes [58]. This recognition is the beginning of a decision to act upon a hazard that has been noticed within the organization, initiating the sensemaking process (*ecological change*).

3.3. Enacting a plan to assess and mitigate risks

After a hazard has been recognized (*ecological change*), any practice that can be used to avoid or minimize risk can be *enacted*. After workplace risk has been recognized (an *ecological change*), they must be assessed and risk control plans that address an organization's unique hazard and risk profiles along with the unique behavioral responses necessary to avoid and/or minimize risk must be developed. These assessments consist of gathering and analyzing safety-relevant information on production processes, machines, equipment, chemicals, workspace layout, existing personnel, laws and regulations, etc. Assessment results should ultimately lead to a thorough understanding of all the hardware and human safety risks the organization is faced with and a plan to help mitigate these risks [57].

3.4. Selecting and executing practices to control risks

At the foundation of ecological change is the recognition that workers who identify H&S hazards are motivated and able to raise their concerns. Tools such as pre-task job briefings, worker self-checking, and stop-think-act-review activities are RM practices that empower and engage workers throughout the sensemaking process [58]. Management, in turn, responds to and engages workers in planning risk mitigation activities. Given limited resources, implementing all possible risk control options may not be feasible [59]. Thus, organizational leaders are usually responsible for choosing an appropriate course of action to reduce the risk (i.e., *selection*). Examples include minimizing physical hazards through proper engineering controls, preventative and predictive maintenance, providing proper equipment, worker training and education, and defining specified patterns of behavior [28].

3.5. Continuous monitoring and retaining outcomes for future risk practices

Finally, the selected action is monitored, assessed, and checked to ensure that the given risk has been minimized to the point of acceptability. Evaluating such efforts could represent both proactive (prior to a safety incident) and reactive (after a safety incident) activities designed to check for workplace hazards and risks that were overlooked or not accurately assessed, or that emerged because of a breakdown in executing certain activities [18, 59]. Examples of *checking* include hazard inspections or audits (proactive checking), and incident investigations (reactive checking) [28]. Risk control practices that successfully reduce uncertainty warrant *retention* of the decision for future use. However, if residual risk is unacceptable, the organization can collectively act to change the initially selected risk control activities. **Figure 2** illustrates how sensemaking can occur parsimoniously within the identification, decision-making, and implementation of the RM cycle.

Figure 2 is depicted to show how the four steps of the sensemaking process can be integrated with the RM cycle to foster an understanding of how to more completely implement an organization's risk management system and continually improve upon it. This integration, however, illuminates the futility of attempts to implement health and safety practices without the necessary organizational infrastructure to support the complete and ongoing sensemaking process throughout the cycle. Organizational and RM characteristics should be structured to support the cognitive, social coordination, and motivational needs that underlie complete sensemaking throughout the cycle. In the following section we discuss these characteristics while continuing to provide general examples of practices within high-risk industries (i.e., mining and construction).

4. Components that facilitate sensemaking

Sensemaking around a consistent organizational RM framework should facilitate a clearer understanding of risks and form a collective sense of what is expected of employees on the job and why. A complete sensemaking process around RM should create a unifying order of how things typically work within the organization. However, if risk practices are not clear and the associated values within an organization are not conducive, employees may not be afforded the opportunity to openly participate in the sensemaking process. The four sensemaking components discussed previously highlight conditions necessary for complete sensemaking around health and safety issues in the workplace to occur. Based on how leaders deliver specific information or lead activities, the organization can be perceived as having various procedures, rites and rituals [60]. Without similar commitment to the organization's goals, workers may have disparate perceptions [61]. Engaging in complete and ongoing sensemaking of H&S risks may help develop and maintain individuals' cognitive, social coordinative, and motivational components needed to accurately perceive and participate in risk management.

4.1. Risk communication to enhance workers' cognitive components

Developing and fostering cognitive components are necessary to facilitate workers' consistent identification of workplace risks, understand the practices necessary to mitigate those risks, and have the efficacy to execute risk practices [62]. Sensemaking, described as "organizing through communication" — can be a helpful alignment process ([63], p. 137). Sensemaking has been shown to help individuals respond to organizational risks or events to prevent workplace accidents [64], demonstrating support for enhanced worker cognition. According to Dixon [65] to "make sense" is not to find the right or wrong answer, but to find a pattern that helps give specific events meaning and direction to the individual, group, or organization. Engaging workers so they have the ability to perceive and initiate responsibility, regardless of the risk, is essential to managing a dynamic environment.

4.2. Risk communication to enhance workers' motivational components

Equally crucial to the consistent communication and interpretation of risks, however, are workers' motivation to execute behaviors needed to prevent an incident. Workers need to believe that if they carry out the desired, or necessary behaviors by way of certain RM practices, they will avoid a negative consequence or receive a positive consequence [10, 12, 14]. However, communication alone is not likely to impact everyone's risk assessment and motivation. In response, a primary task of top-level leadership is to create an organizational culture that values and rewards assessment and communication pertaining to risk-related events [66].

Organizations can use sensemaking processes to help facilitate a more organized, communicative process that involves the interpretation of events in the environment, social interactions to interpret those events, and constructing the responses necessary to mitigate a problem or improve a process [67, 68]. Along these same lines, a social component is necessary regarding, namely the importance of everyone being on the same page both cognitively and motivationally. More specifically, because risk mitigation often depends on the collective work unit and because the work is increasingly interdependent, it is important for everyone to establish a common perception of, agreement about, and response to workplace risks [63].

4.3. Designing risk communication

Based on a review of the organizational psychology and strategic management literature, we suggest that sensemaking around risk management should be structured so that three interrelated characteristics are clearly illustrated to employees: (1) Distinctiveness; (2) Consistency; and (3) Consensus. These three characteristics have been theoretically associated with having positive effects on the strength of sensemaking primarily by enhancing vertical and horizontal trust within the organization, thereby facilitating the open flow of critical information and in turn facilitating the implementation of organizational management systems [68–70]. We argue that these three characteristics are prerequisites of vertical and horizontal trust around H&S issues. We further suggest that this enhanced sensemaking leads to the consistent execution of routine H&S behaviors and the ability to manage risks in dynamic and uncertain contexts. **Figure 3** illustrates this model.

4.3.1. Message distinctiveness

Distinctiveness refers to the features of the practices that facilitate the execution of desired activities to stand out in the workplace, while capturing the attention and interest of workers [69]. These authors state that visibility is a "basic prerequisite for interpretation involving whether a practice and its component parts are disclosed to employees, affording them the opportunity for sensemaking" (p. 208). Visibility is a fundamental component for how workers attend to and organize risk-based information on the job. Unclear aspects of these practices could influence what risks workers choose to pay attention to (i.e., enact), and how they respond (i.e., select). A distinctive system also fosters well-understood values and associated practices by workers [69]. If workers do not understand particular H&S risk practices, they will not know which choices (i.e., selections) are shared among the organization and, potentially misunderstand why certain behavioral responses may be desired and how to execute these practices. Alternatively, conscious and open sensemaking conversations function as a sense of empowerment for workers, because they can identify and respond to smaller incidents in an effort to prevent larger problems [65].

Features of distinctiveness highlight the importance of communication to increase accuracy and uniformity in message interpretation. All risk communication should be visible and understandable between managers and workers to allow personal experience at both levels to be incorporated into selecting and retaining best practices [11]. In this regard, risk communication

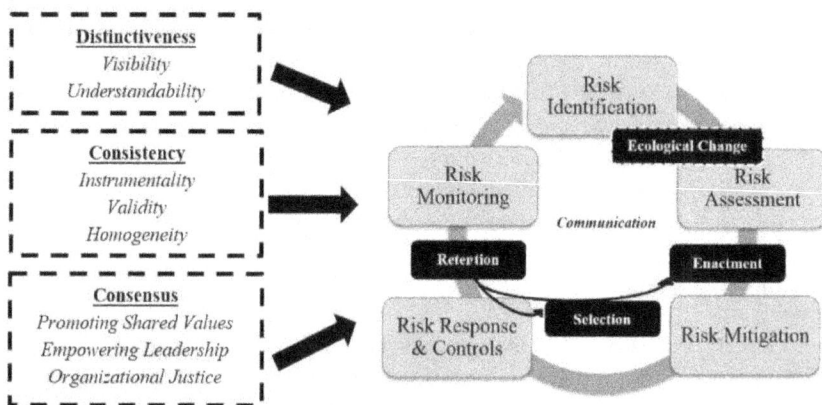

Figure 3. Characteristics of risk communication that facilitate sensemaking.

theories can guide and improve message distinctiveness within organizations to help motivate appropriate behavioral responses. For example, gain and loss-framed messages can be used to persuade a desired response, depending on whether or not the group responds better to a negatively or positively valenced message [71].

4.3.2. Message consistency

Consistency is established over time when the same outcome occurs in response to the same incident [70]. Sensemaking is also contingent upon what is consistently reinforced, expected, rewarded, and reprimanded within the organization [71]. Additionally, from a risk communication perspective, including normative language helps an organization's survival and strategic adoption to crises over time [70]. Several features of consistency exist. First, *instrumentality* encompasses a clear, "perceived cause-effect relationship in reference to the management systems' desired content-focused behaviors and associated employee consequences" (p. 210). Workers' perception of the organization's instrumentality is formed by reinforcement and repetition of messages and outcomes over time [47, 69]. Therefore, reinforcement of desired H&S practices may be better achieved when an organization has a strong internal communication system with built-in redundancies [4]. As a result, similar incentives and consequences associated with workers' selection, or decision-making within the organization, may improve workers' motivation to participate in the RM cycle.

Additionally, to foster consistency within the organization, it is important to consider and communicate the validity of each H&S practice desired by the organization. System practices must exhibit consistency between what they intend to do and what they actually do [69]. If an ecological change occurs that is not perceived as relevant, enactment on behalf of an individual may not occur. This premise suggests that mandated H&S behaviors incorporated into activities must be explicitly relevant to actual risk presented by work processes. If workers are not able to make a cognitive connection between a given H&S practice that they are expected to perform and the outcomes promised by the organization, then the message to workers is potentially contradictory and inconsistent with the purpose of the practice. As a result, enactment and selection of what these workers pay attention to may change over time.

Contradictory practices included within an organization's strategic goals undermine its structural consistency. Internal alignment and support of RM practices help workers perceive consistent values of the organization and thus, respond appropriately during an ecological change. For example, if certain skills are given priority during training of new employees, these same types of skills should be observed and rewarded on the job so workers understand and see the importance of transferring these skills to on the job tasks in an effort to mitigate identified risks during the training.

Finally, the structural characteristic of consistency can be influenced by what the various organizational decision makers pay attention and respond to each day [55]. In order for the RM process to be consistent, communication and coordination among various levels of organizational management is crucial. Heterogeneity across organizational leaders in the reinforcement of which types of health and safety behaviors are important undermines HSMS consistency. Therefore, managers must relay the same message to the workers on each shift so the organization's goals and values are consistent, regardless of who is communicating at the time. Workers' communication is both enabled and constrained by the values that make up the culture of an organization [4]. For sensemaking to be effective in workplace safety, the culture of the organization has to be conducive to unimpeded information flow such as the reporting of near misses and other risky events noticed [72]. Impediments to free-flowing communication in this case may consist of fear of management reprisal or co-worker judgment [54, 56]. Therefore, fostering an environment free of negative consequences by peers and managers, is an important feature needed for sensemaking.

4.3.3. Message consensus

Finally, the structural characteristic of consistency can be influenced by what the various organizational decision-makers pay attention and respond to each day [55]. *Consensus* is agreement among workers, as to what H&S practices, and their associated behaviors, lead to intended organizational outcomes (e.g., reduction in H&S incidents) [69, 70]. Achieving consensus on an individual and organizational level can be difficult, but is critical for organizational function [73]. Because sensemaking is best facilitated through a just culture with strong organizational values, shared values and worker involvement are important to establishing site-wide consensus. Consensus requires competent leaders who are willing to engage in open dialog with workers. In response, leaders' sensegiving should possess intuition, logic, emotional intelligence, self-awareness, inductive/deductive reasoning, and the ability to look for and provide strategic evidence to support the RM decisions made [63]. In addition, it is important to know if workers perceive the organization to be fair and just. Perceived fairness is associated with workers' attitudes and behaviors as well as influences their acceptance of the H&S practices, rules, and regulations they are expected to follow [74].

4.4. Bringing it all together

Albeit this theoretical integration appears complex, in practice this process serves to reduce ambiguity encountered through unexpected, potentially risky events and near misses, which occur daily by rank-and-file workers in high-risk jobs. Because sensemaking is an active process of assigning meaning, it can only occur through human reflection [45]. Within this chapter, we argued that this reflection can occur best if organized and presented through the risk management process, along with joint participation from hourly workers and their management. To put this argument into practice, consider the following example on a job site:

Sensemaking is initially triggered by a situation that creates ambiguity for the worker—take for example a key piece of machinery experiencing problems that may make it unsafe to operate. This malfunction occurs while employees have a high work order they are in the process of filling—with the deadline for shipment fast approaching. This occurrence is likely to cause a discrepancy between what management expects and what the workers experience. This breakdown initiates enactment on behalf of the workers, triggering a risk assessment about whether or not to keep running the machine. In this case, the worker may choose to consult the job task analysis for the piece of machinery, consult a coworker who is in the maintenance department, or contact management for next steps. These assessment results should help minimize ambiguity and lead to a thorough understanding of the potential risks if the site keeps operating with the equipment. Based on this information, the workforce can select an appropriate course of action to minimize the risks—whether it includes providing additional protection for workers who operate the machine, putting a new engineering control in place, or stopping production for fix the machine.

Whatever action is selected, the sensemaking process continues with monitoring and assessing if the risk was controlled appropriately to see if the decision should be retained. Although this example is hypothetical, we can all glean that stopping production would be the safest, least risky option for the workforce, even if it means production and delivery obligations temporarily suffer. This is when the concepts of organizational messaging discussed in the chapter become critical for reducing ambiguity. If messages received by the workers from their management up to this point have been distinctive, consistent, and encompass justice and shared values, coming to this decision is expected to be easier by the workers involved in this uncertain situation.

For example, if distinctive communication had been fostered by management, workers should know how to attend to and organize these unexpected events on the job—meaning they would interpret the situation as a risk and understand that immediate action was needed. In response, if management does not actively provide visible priorities to their workers, they should reassess current modes of communication to ensure that safety is a priority over production. This concept flows into the consistency of such messaging as well. Even though some modes of communication may visibly show this priority, management has to be on board and consistently say and support this same message. Therefore, if a worker had received praise for going around a risky situation in the past to meet a production goal, it is likely this worker would do the same thing (i.e., retained the same action in their last sensemaking for future use). However, if this action received negative consequences, then a different, safer option would be selected. Therefore, all managers must support the same actions among their workforce, not just one. This consistency also helps foster consensus on the job site, establishing the same health and safety goals for both workers and management [69].

5. Conclusion

This chapter focused on the barriers to RM and potential benefits of both leaders and workers engaging in sensemaking processes to help deliver, influence, interpret and execute desired RM practices. This integrated, cyclical system may result in the following: (1) workers may be more confident in and committed to the organization due to a more accurate interpretation of their work environment; (2) workers may share the same interpretation of what is important, expected, and rewarded in that environment; and (3) workers may be more interested in helping the organization achieve its strategic goals [69]. Therefore, sensemaking can be viewed as a RM process which allows everyone to identify hazards, communicate about the risks, and respond accordingly. Although the communicators within the system are key players in fostering consensus and fairness in the system, how organizations progress through structural communication barriers remains a challenge [71]. If we can better identify and understand tangible behaviors of organizational leaders that are perceived as positive and encourage worker engagement, it may be easier to support organizations in improving structural deficiencies and eventually, execute a consistent health and safety management system to predict, identify, and mitigate risks.

Conflict of interest

Replace the entirety of this text with the 'conflict of interest' declaration.

Author details

Emily J. Haas[1*] and Patrick L. Yorio[2]

*Address all correspondence to: ejhaas@cdc.gov

1 National Institute for Occupational Safety and Health, Pittsburgh Mining Research Division, Pittsburgh, PA, USA

2 National Institute for Occupational Safety and Health, National Personal Protective Technology Laboratory, Pittsburgh, PA, USA

References

[1] Boyle T. Health and Safety: Risk Management. New York: Routledge; 2012

[2] Frick K, Wren J. Reviewing Occupational Health and Safety Management: Multiple Roots, Diverse Perspectives and Ambiguous Outcomes. Systematic Occupational Health and Safety Management: Perspectives and International Development. Amsterdan: Pergamon; 2000. pp. 17-42

[3] Guidotti TL. Communication models in environmental health. Journal of Health Communication. 2013;**18**:66-79

[4] Keyton J. Communication and Organizational Culture: A Key to Understanding Work Experiences. 2nd ed. Thousand Oaks: Sage; 2011

[5] Barling J, Hutchinson I. Commitment vs. control-based safety practices, safety reputation, and perceived safety climate. Canadian Journal of Administrative Sciences. 2000; **28**:76-84

[6] Hofmann DA, Morgeson FP. Safety-related behavior as a social exchange: The role of perceived organizational support and leader–member exchange. The Journal of Applied Psychology. 1999;**84**:286

[7] Zacharatos A, Barling J, Iverson RD. High-performance work systems and occupational safety. The Journal of Applied Psychology. 2005;**90**:77

[8]   Zohar D. Modifying supervisory practices to improve subunit safety: A leadership-based intervention model. The Journal of Applied Psychology. 2002;**87**:156-163

[9]   Zohar D, Luria G. The use supervisory practices as leverage to improve safety behavior: A cross-level intervention model. Journal of Safety Research. 2003;**34**:567-577

[10]   Zohar D, Polachek T. Discourse-based intervention for modifying supervisory communication as leverage for safety climate and performance improvement: A randomized field study. The Journal of Applied Psychology. 2014;**99**:113-124

[11]   Hale A, Borys D. Working to rule, or working safely? Part 1: A state of the art review. Safety Science. 2013;**55**:207-221

[12]   Hofmann DA, Morgeson FP, Gerras SJ. Climate as a moderator of the relationship between leader-member exchange and content specific citizenship: Safety climate as an exemplar. The Journal of Applied Psychology. 2003;**88**:170

[13]   Hofmann DA, Stetzer A. The role of safety climate and communication in accident interpretation: Implications for learning from negative events. Academy of Management Journal. 1998;**41**:644-657

[14]   Christian MS, Bradley JC, Wallace JC, Burke MJ. Workplace safety: A meta-analysis of the roles of person and situation factors. The Journal of Applied Psychology. 2009;**94**:1102-1127

[15]   Griffin MA, Parker SK, Mason CM. Leader vision and the development of adaptive and proactive performance: A longitudinal study. The Journal of Applied Psychology. 2010;**95**:174

[16]   Griffin MA, Neal A, Parker SK. A new model of work role performance: Positive behavior in uncertain and interdependent contexts. Academy of Management Journal. 2007;**50**:327-347

[17]   Dohmen T, Falk A, Huffman D, Sunde U, Schupp J, Wagner GG. Individual risk attitudes: Measurement, determinants, and behavioral consequences. Journal of the European Economic Association. 2011;**9**:522-550

[18]   DeJoy DM, Schaffer BS, Wilson MG, Vandenberg RJ, Butts MM. Creating safer workplaces: Assessing the determinants and role of safety climate. Journal of Safety Research. 2004;**35**:81-90

[19]   Flach JM, Carroll JS, Dainoff MJ, Hamilton WI. Striving for safety: Communicating and deciding in sociotechnical systems. Ergonomics. 2015;**58**:615-634

[20]   Yorio PL, Willmer DR, Moore SM. Management systems through a multilevel and strategic management perspective: Theoretical and empirical considerations. Safety Science. 2015;**72**:221-228

[21]   Zohar D. Safety climate and beyond: A multi-level multi-climate framework. Safety Science. 2008;**46**:376-387

[22] Kirsch P, Hine A, Maybury T. A model for the implementation of industry-wide knowledge sharing to improve risk management practice. Safety Science. 2015;**80**:66-76

[23] Robson LS et al. The effectiveness of occupational health and safety management system interventions: A systematic review. Safety Science. 2007;**45**:329-353

[24] Baker S, Ponniah D, Smith S. Risk response techniques employed currently for major projects. Construction Management and Economics. 1999;**17**:205-213

[25] Boehm BW. Software Risk Management. Piscataway, NJ: IEEE Press; 1989

[26] British Standards Institution. Occupational health and safety management systems – Specification, BS OHSAS 18001; 2007

[27] Smith SP, Harrison MD. Measuring reuse in hazard analysis. Reliability Engineering and System Safety. 2005;**89**:93

[28] Haas EJ, Yorio P. Exploring the state of health and safety management system performance measurement in mining organizations. Safety Science. 2016;**83**:48-58

[29] Janicak CA. Safety Metrics: Tools and Techniques for Measuring Safety Performance. 2nd ed. Lantham, MD: Scarecrow Press; 2011. Government Institutes

[30] Makin AM, Winder C. A new conceptual framework to improve the application of occupational health and safety management systems. Safety Science. 2008;**46**:935-948

[31] Brassell-Cicchinit LA. The shareholder value of crisis handling. Risk Management. 2003; **50**:48

[32] Covello VT. Risk communication: An emerging area of health communication research. In: Deetz SA, editor. Communication Yearbook. Newbury Park, CA: Sage; 1992

[33] Cuny X, Lejeune M. Statistical modelling & risk assessment. Safety Science. 2003;**41**:29

[34] McComas KA. Defining moments in risk communication research: 1996-2005. Journal of Health Communication. 2006;**11**:75-91

[35] Palenchar MJ. Risk communication. In: Heath RL, editor. Encyclopedia of Public Relations. Thousand Oaks, CA: Sage; 2005. pp. 752-755

[36] Coombs WT. Ongoing Crisis Communication: Planning, Managing, and Responding. 3rd ed. Thousand Oaks, CA: Sage; 2012

[37] Brun W. Cognitive components in risk perception: Natural versus manmade risks. Journal of Behavioral Decision Making. 1992;**5**:117-132

[38] Reason J. A Life in Error: From Little Slips to Big Disasters. Burlington, VT: Ashgate Publishing; 2013

[39] Weinstein ND. Optimistic biases about personal risks. Science. 1989;**246**:1232-1233

[40] Zohar D, Erev I. On the difficulty of promoting workers' safety behaviour: Overcoming the underweighting of routine risks. International Journal of Risk Assessment and Management. 2006;**7**:122-136

[41] Haas E, Mattson M. A qualitative comparison of susceptibility and behavior in recreational and occupational risk environments: Implications for promoting health and safety. Journal of Health Communication. 2016. DOI: 10.1080/10810730.2016.1153765

[42] Reason J. Achieving a safe culture: Theory and practice. Work and Stress. 1998;**12**:293-306

[43] Wold T, Laumann K. Safety management systems as communication in an oil and gas producing company. Safety Science. 2015;**72**:23-30

[44] Neal A, Griffin MA. Safety climate and safety behavior. Journal of Management. 2002;**27**:67-75

[45] Battles JB, Dixon NM, Borotkanics RJ, Rabin-Fastmen B, Kaplan HS. Sensemaking of patient safety risks and hazards. Health Services Research. 2006;**41**:1555-1575

[46] DeRosier J, Stalhandske E, Bagian JP, Nudell T. Using health care failure mode and effect analysis: The VA national center for patient safety's prospective risk analysis system. The Joint Commission Journal on Quality Improvement. 2002;**28**:248-267

[47] Weick KE. The reduction of medical errors through mindful interdependence. In: Rosenthal MM, Sutcliffe KM, editors. Medical Error: What Do we Know? What Do we Do? San Francisco, CA: Jossey-Bass; 2002

[48] Wreathall J, Nemeth C. Assessing risk: The role of probabilistic risk assessment (PRA) in patient safety improvement. Quality & Safety in Health Care. 2004;**13**:206-212

[49] van Tonder C, Groenwald JP. Of mining accidents and sense-making: Traversing well-trodden ground. Journal of Global Business and Technology. 2001;**7**:57-73

[50] Weick KE. The collapse of sensemaking in organizations: The Man Gulch disaster. Administrative Science Quarterly. 1993;**38**:100-124

[51] Bartunek JM, Krim RM, Necochea R, Humphries M. Sensemaking, sensegiving, and leadership in strategic organizational development. Advances in Qualitative Organizational Research. 1999;**2**:37-71

[52] Battles JB, Lilford RJ. Organizing patient safety research to identify risks and hazards. Quality & Safety in Health Care. 2003;**12**(Suppl II):ii2-ii7

[53] Weick KE. Sensemaking in Organizations. Thousand Oaks, CA: Sage; 1995

[54] Weick KE. The Psychology of Organizing. 2nd ed. Reading, MA: Addison-Wesley; 1979

[55] Millar DP, Heath RL. A rhetorical approach to crisis communication: Management, communication processes, and strategic responses. In: Millar DP, Heath RL, editors. Responding to Crisis: A Rhetorical Approach to Crisis Communication. Mahwah, NJ: Lawrence Erlbaum; 2004

[56] Seeger MW, Sellnow TL, Ulmer RR. Communication, organization and crisis. In: Roloff ME, editor. Communication Yearbook 21. Thousand Oaks, CA: Sage; 1998

[57] Yorio PL, Willmer DR, Haight JM. Interpreting MSHA citations through the lens of occupational health and safety management systems: Investigating their impact on mine injuries and illnesses 2003-2010. Risk Analysis. 2014;**34**:1538-1553

[58] Wachter JK, Yorio PL. Human performance tools: Engaging workers as the best defense against errors and their precursors. Professional Safety. 2013;**59**:54-64

[59] Stephans RA. System Safety for the 21st Century: The Updated and Revised Edition of System Safety. Hoboken, New Jersey: John Wiley & Sons; 2012

[60] Schein EH. Organizational Culture and Leadership. San Francisco, CA: Jossey-Bass; 1992

[61] Foldy EG, Goldman L, Ospina S. Sensegiving and the role of cognitive shifts in the work of leadership. The Leadership Quarterly. 2008;**19**:514-529

[62] Barrick MR, Mount MK. Yes, personality matters: Moving on to more important matters. Human Performance. 2005;**18**:359-372

[63] Weick KE, Sutcliffe KM, Obstfeld D. Organizing and the process of sensemaking. Organization Science. 2005;**16**:409-421

[64] Gephart RP. The textual approach: Risk and blame in disaster sensemaking. The Academy of Management Journal. 1993;**36**:1465-1514

[65] Dixon NM. Sensemaking Guidelines – A Quality Improvement Tool. Med QIC Medicare Quality Improvement. Baltimore: Centers of Medicare and Medicaid Services; 2003

[66] Clarke S, Ward K. The role of leader influence tactics and safety climate in engaging employee's safety participation. Risk Analysis. 2006;**26**:1175-1185

[67] Judge TA, Bono JE. Five factor model of personality and transformational leadership. The Journal of Applied Psychology. 2000;**85**:751-765

[68] Wardman JK. The constitution of risk communication in advanced liberal societies. Risk Analysis. 2008;**28**:1619-1637

[69] Bowen DE, Ostroff C. Understanding HRM-firm performance linkages: The role of the "strength" of the HRM system. Academy of Management. 2004;**29**:203-221

[70] Kelley HH. The processes of causal attribution. The American Psychologist. 1973;**28**: 107-128

[71] Cho H. Health Communication Message Design. Thousand Oaks, CA: Sage; 2012

[72] Marx D. Patient Safety and the "Just Culture": A Primer for Health Care Executives. New York: Columbia University; 2001

[73] Vancouver JB, Schmitt NW. An exploratory examination of person-organization fit: Organizational goal congruence. Personnel Psychology. 1991;**44**:333-352

[74] Bretz RD, Milkovich GT, Read W. The state of performance appraisal research and practice: Concerns, directions, and implications. Journal of Management. 1992;**18**:321-352

Healthcare Message Design toward Social Communication: Convergence Based on Philosophical and Theoretical Perspectives

Ji-Young An and Jinkyung Paik

Additional information is available at the end of the chapter

http://dx.doi.org/10.5772/intechopen.76254

Abstract

The importance of communication in healthcare has gained considerable attention especially with the rise of the model of patient-centered care. There are many types of messages between healthcare providers and consumers, which is an intangible form of healthcare message design (HMD) as a medium of communication. In the role, HMD is understood as an expansion of universal communicability and plays an important role in social communication. This chapter introduces the concept of HMD based on philosophical underpinnings and theoretical frameworks and defines the process of HMD. For the work, convergence research (or transdisciplinarity, and interdisciplinarity) was conducted, which entails integrating knowledge, theories, methods, data, and expertise from different disciplines.

Keywords: communication, convergence, interdisciplinarity, empathy, healthcare, nursing, philosophy, relationship, theory, transdisciplinarity

1. Introduction

Health is defined as a state of complete physical, social, and mental well-being and not merely the absence of illness, disease, or infirmity [1, 2]. Sociologist Aaron Antonovsky (1923–1994), the father of the *salutogenesis*, interpreted health as a "sense of coherence" or "becoming" rather than "being." Health (*salus*) is continuously being generated (*genesis*) [3]. Individual health is not fixed or static but requires continuous effort to maintain the status of "being healthy" in the process of change to protect against disease or injury. Healthcare is defined as "the organized provision of medical care to individuals or a community" [4]. Continuous health-care focuses not on the treatment of disease but on the continuum of health management for curing, recovering, and healing through medical treatment, nursing, and caring throughout an individual's entire life within the systematic structure [5, 6]. In the provision of such services, communication between consumers and providers should be empathetic [2, 4]. Furthermore, there should be a strong social awareness of public healthcare services that are available. Therapeutic interactions through empathy make it possible to have insight into another person's thoughts or feelings, which, as we shall see, is vital to *salutogenic* healthcare [7, 8].

It is necessary for consumers to efficiently communicate with their healthcare providers in a safe, reliable, and informative way. Previous studies have reported that design should play an integral part in facilitating communication [6, 9, 10]. Recently, convergence research (or transdisciplinarity, interdisciplinarity) has been vigorously pushed forward [11], which entails integrating knowledge, theories, methods, data, and expertise from different disciplines and forming new frameworks, paradigms, or even disciplines to catalyze innovation across multiple research communities [6, 10, 11]. Healthcare design as a newly emerging discipline is an example of this approach, which focuses on therapeutic interactions between space and behavior for creating healing environments and improving health outcomes [6, 9, 10, 12, 13].

The importance of communication in healthcare has gained considerable attention especially with the rise of the concept of patient-centered care [14–17]. The patient-centered care model [16] stresses elements of health communication such as open-ended inquiry, reflective listening, empathy, and the identity (values and preferences) of individuals [17]. Designing messages effectively can serve as a medium of social communication [6, 10]. The goal of this interdisciplinary effort is to integrate design into health communication. Healthcare message design (HMD) is a new concept that needs to be defined philosophically and theoretically, which blends scientific disciplines in a coordinated, reciprocal way *to* develop effective ways of communicating across disciplines by adopting common frameworks and a new scientific language. This chapter introduces the concept of HMD based on philosophical underpinnings and theoretical frameworks and defines the process of HMD, which encompasses information, sustainability, partnership, publicness, integrity, and health promotion [6, 10]. Practically, it is expected that the content discussed in this chapter can provide a basis for future research on the implementation of HMD toward social communication.

2. Conceptual framework

This proposed conceptual framework is a modified hybrid model (**Figure 1**), which was based on the work proposed by Kim et al. [18, 19] and Parse's human-becoming theory [20]. The model consists of three interrelated phases: a theoretical phase, a fieldwork phase, and a final analytical phase. In this chapter, only the theoretical phase of this framework was adapted to theoretically define the concept of HMD, which consists of the following four attributes: concepts (healthcare, design, and communication), an interdisciplinary approach, meanings and measurements, and working conditions. The fieldwork phase and the final analytical phase will not be discussed because of the scope of this study.

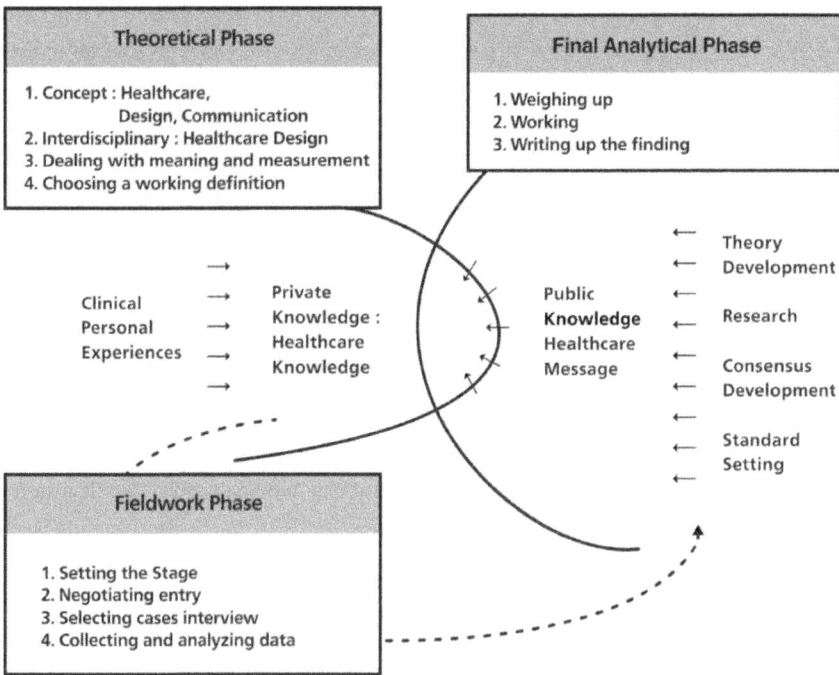

Figure 1. Conceptual framework.

3. Healthcare message design

Communication means (1) information exchange by speaking, writing, or using some other medium, (2) the successful conveying or sharing of ideas and feelings, and (3) social contact by means of sending or receiving information [21]. Immanuel Kant (1724–1804) provided the philosophical premise of communication and proposed the concept of *ästhetische Kommunikation* in the *Critique of Judgment* [22, 23]. *Social communication of beauty* should include not only the other but also the self; thereby, a social sharing of emotion is possible. Previous research has focused on efficient communication between providers and consumers fostered through mutual empathy [24, 25]. Emmanuel Lévinas stated, "The *Subject* is absorbed in the object it absorbs, and nevertheless keeps a distance" [26]. He also defined "the *Other* [as] an absolutely different person." Lévinas added that the Object is represented to the Subject as a painful face deprived of everything.

Empathy, which is the ability to understand the others in their experience, can make communication easier through a shared metaphor such as *beauty* or design [8, 22]. The philosophical underpinnings of empathy date back to Kant, who related empathy to the universal sense of *beauty* between the Subject and the Object [22, 23]. Kant utilized the term *Gemeinsinn* (*sensus communis*) to describe the universal sharing of the sense of *beauty*. *Ästhetischer Gemeinsinn* (*sensus communis aestheticus*), referred to by Kant as *ästhetische Kommunikation* [23], made an individual feel *beauty*, and because *beauty* is universal, an individual is able to reach into the realm of universal thought. *Ästhetischer Gemeinsinn*, in other words, is a subjective condition of *universal communicability*. In the *Critique of Judgment* [22], universal communicability was viewed as social esthetics. The term "universal" includes both the Subject and the Object; thus, universal communicability can actualize the body of social communication by an individual's choice in public sphere [6]. Social communication is possible when there is freedom to assert one's thought in the public domain while recognizing the differences of others [23].

Philosophy recognizes empathy as the extension of image schemata and expands the concept to include the other within oneself who recognizes others as different from oneself [26]. Bodily pain is "a complex social and psychological entity" beyond the pain [27]. Communication that delivers messages regarding human dignity and the value of life can be considered an important medium of artistic nursing [28]. Decision making for self-care is essentially based on informed decisions; therefore, information is essential to the improvement of health outcomes. Consumers gain power and confidence by actively participating in their care according to accurate and reliable information. Therefore, there is a need to design health communication that effectively delivers information.

Especially in the discipline of nursing, which is based on the philosophical understanding of a person as a whole, Carl Rogers [29] defined empathy as "being able to perceive another's feelings and experiences with accuracy." It has also been reported that empathy is one of the most important characteristics for aiding therapeutic relationships [7, 24, 30]. Florence Nightingale (1820–1910) actualized the concept of empathy by addressing social and psychological environment including chattering hopes and advices, and petty management. Nightingale defined "petty management" of the other as the Object in the community; in other words, "by not knowing how to manage that what you do when you are there, shall be done when you are not there" [31].

The importance of empathy has been introduced as a core of common aims within a conceptual framework for health professionals [32, 33]. Empathy is a core competence of healthcare providers; however, the concept of empathy seems to be still complex and multidimensional [7, 34–36]. Theoretically, it is assumed that empathy plays a role in healthcare providers' performance, which is related to patient satisfaction or even patient compliance, patient enablement, and clinical outcomes [14, 24, 30, 37, 38]. Empathy has three different competencies such as an affective attitude (compassionate care), a cognitive skill (perspective taking), and communicative behaviors, which provide insight into others' thoughts and emotions [7, 30, 32].

For the philosophical understanding of communication in health care, the awareness of oneself and others originates in philosophy. According to Kant, there is a kind of shared meaning that is not reducible to conceptual and propositional content alone [22, 23]. This insight was expanded by Mark Johnson who proposed that such thought is pre-conceptual and involves the metaphoric extension of image schemata, which means the acknowledgement of the distance between each other [39]. The Object cannot be the cognitive possession of the Subject nor recognized as the same as oneself (the Subject) when recognized as the Object.

The scope of health communication covers "disease control and prevention, emergency preparedness and response, injury and violence prevention, environmental health, and workplace safety and health" [40]. Patient-centered communication based on empathy has demonstrated clinically positive effects on patient outcomes such as satisfaction, compliance, and diagnosis or treatment [16, 17]. For example, Wanzer et al. stressed that empathy in particular can reduce patients' anxiety [14]. Fox et al. reported that doctors who had experienced serious health problems felt more empathy when they communicated with their patients and especially showed more empathy when communicating with patients who had similar health problems to theirs [24].

Origins of design are the Latin *disegno* and *designare*. *Disegno*, or *desseing*, means "a plan to draw a picture." This originates in the division made in *Trattato di pittura* (1509) by the sixteenth-century painter Lancilotti, who said that the characteristics of painting consisted of *disegno, colorito, compositione*, and *inventione*. Therefore, the meaning of *disegno* is akin to the dictionary definition of "plan" [41], and its meaning has been expanded to include creative thinking, which is working in an artist's mind. *Designare* is a compound word using the prefix, *de*, and the root word, *signare*. *De* means to take away and *signare* means sign or symbol. Combining these two meanings, *designare* has been expanded beyond the primary dictionary meaning of symbol or sign to include the meaning of "meta," which is the interpretation and creation of cultural symbols as well [42]. In this sense, design can be described as an effort to create a meaningful order in human behavior [43].

In healthcare, design plays a meaningful role throughout the entire therapeutic and or healing process that is "other-centered "or "audience-centered" caring and the consideration of other people's circumstances [44]. Design in healthcare as an integrated practice of empathic design results in healthcare systems that place an increased value on the patient's engagement in care process [45, 46]. Designing healthcare systems requires a deep understanding of care protocols, patient safety, and efficacy requirements, user needs and experience, environmental and technological contexts, and organizational behaviors [12, 13, 45–48]. Ulrich [12] focused on psychosocial support in creating a healing environment that maintains and improves the status of health, namely supportive design [13]. The approach of design in healthcare unifies theories and practices by focusing on human experience that redefines healthcare design and patient care [49].

In this context, designing is the shared metaphor that enables individuals to understand the emotions of others. Designing health communication is a progress of signifying practice through the intervention of design. For designing messages in health communication, empathy of consumer's various tastes and preferences should be taken into consideration by healthcare professionals. To that end, it should be based on a certain degree of philosophical premise to the other within oneself. In other words, HMD represents the experiences of the Subject and the Object as a shared metaphor formulating empathy between providers and consumers. As a result, HMD can play an important mediatory role in enhancing health outcomes and simultaneously facilitate the therapeutic and or healing process when it is approached through the meta-concept based on social esthetics.

4. Theoretical framework

To propose a theoretical framework of HMD, Parse's ground theory of human becoming was borrowed, which encompasses three major themes: meaning, rhythmicity, and co-transcendence [20]. The theory of human becoming was developed to move nursing's view of a person from a medical model to a human science [50]. In the theory, the person is seen as "a participant in experiencing situations." The theory explains "how the meaning in any situation is related to the particular constituents of that situation" [51]. Parse emphasized that a human being can become human becoming by exchanging energies through interaction between other human beings and their environment [52–54].

Parse identified nine themes from the three philosophical assumptions (**Table 1**). In the theory, "meaning" refers to an ever-changing interpretation one gives to what is valued and the ways in which these interpretations reflect the person's reality. "Rhythmicity" refers to the cadent, mutual patterning of the human-universe mutual process. "Transcendence" refers to reaching beyond the possible, to the hopes and dreams envisioned in multidimensional experiences [20, 50, 52].

Human becoming is (1) freely choosing personal meaning in situations in the inter-subjective process of living value priorities, (2) co-creating rhythmical patterns of relating in mutual process with the universe, and (3) co-transcending multidimensionally with the emerging possible [20, 51, 54, 55]. **Figure 2** presents the concept of HMD based on these philosophical principles as a medium of communication within the health information context.

In this context (**Figure 2**), "meaning" is the effort to create an other-centered environment with the view that human care and the healthcare environment are not fixed; therefore, the other is an individual entity as a whole (illuminating meaning of others' experience). "Rhythmicity" is the development of partnership through openness of environment, that is, the development of empathy through continuous relationship with others (concurrently synchronizing rhythms for patients and their family members or caregivers). "Co-transcendence" is infinite potentiality to expand empathy, strengthening one's own specific method and mobilizing transcendence, reaching beyond and transforming toward possibility.

The ultimate product of HMD is better health outcomes, which facilitate the healing process and human dignity by way of "caring presence" [56]. This is in the same vein with the "ethics of care" based on emotion that is advocated by Carol Gilligan [57], which originates from the premises that (1) as humans, we are inherently relational and responsive beings and (2) the human condition is one of connectedness and interdependences (**Figure 3**). Ethics of care

Nine themes from philosophical assumptions	
Meaning	Imaging, valuing, languaging
Rhythmicity	Revealing-concealing, enabling-limiting, connecting-separating
Co-transcendence	Powering, originating, transforming

Table 1. Three principles of Parse's human-becoming theory.

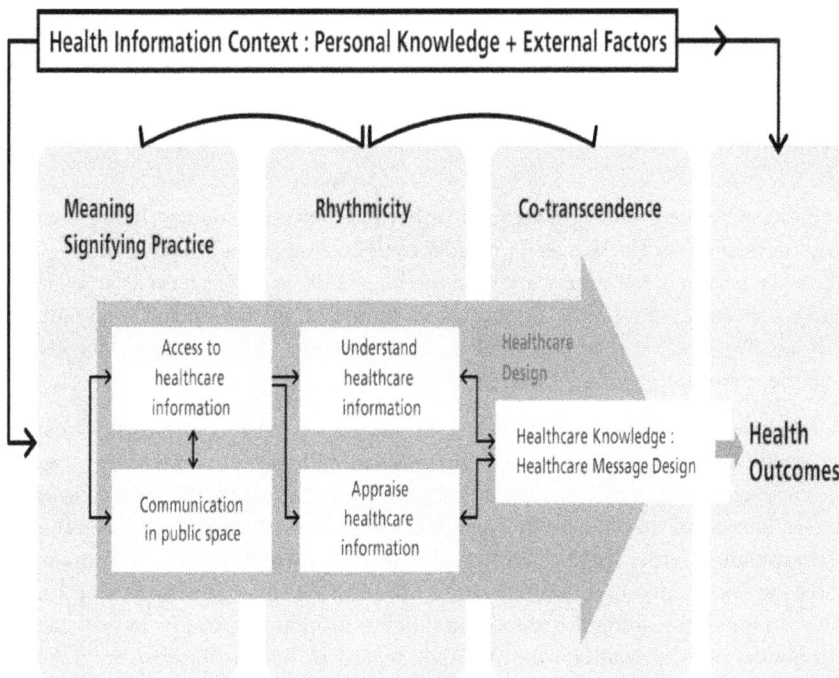

Figure 2. Health information context.

Stage	Principle of Care
Post-Conventional	Principle of nonviolence
Conventional	Self sacrifice for the greater good
Pre- Conventional	Individual survival

Transition from Goodness to Truth

Transition from Selfishness to Responsibility

Figure 3. Ethics of care.

directs our attention to the need for responsiveness in relationships (paying attention, listening, responding) and to the costs of losing connection with oneself or with others. Its logic is inductive, contextual, and psychological, rather than deductive or mathematical.

Current practice establishes providers as advocates for their consumers. For example, pain perceived by patients should be understood not just as a complaint but as a part of agony. This is why medical humanism must embrace the patients' pain [10, 27, 58]. The essence of suffering, as depicted by Eric Cassell, is "experienced by persons, not merely by bodies, and has its source in challenges that threaten the intactness of the person as a complex social and psychological entity" [27]. Parse's theory of human becoming also assists individuals in taking an active decision-making role in self-care, so that patients feel empowered [20, 54].

Accordingly, other-centered or audience-centered HMD highly regards the various channels for communication that makes access to healthcare service consistent [44, 58].

5. Conclusion

Communication delivers messages through verbal and non-verbal means. In healthcare, there are many types of messages between providers and consumers, which is an intangible form of HMD as a medium of communication. In the role, HMD is understood as an expansion of universal communicability [6, 10, 22] and plays an important role in social communication [6, 10, 24, 25, 59]. HMD can be expanded to include a new, shared esthetic sensitivity that *beauty* can be communicated as a social medium [5, 8, 22, 23].

Studies introduced in the *Bulletin*, which is published by the World Health Organization, have reported that communication is a complex social process but contributes to health outcomes (i.e., a major change in health behaviors) [60]. The Institute of Medicine calls upon educators in healthcare for the efficient delivery of patient-centered care through communication [14–17]. In nursing, Carper [61] has advanced four fundamental patterns of knowing; one of these, esthetic knowledge that is often called the *art of nursing*, is subjective and intuition-based. It calls for appreciating the unique qualities of individual patients as well as responding with compassion to facilitate the therapeutic and or healing process for better health outcomes.

In this chapter, to introduce the new concept of HMD, the convergence approach based on philosophical underpinnings and theoretical frameworks was emphasized. The core of HMD should be the understanding of the other within oneself, which can be actualized through the convergence approach regarding healthcare, design, and communication. Therefore, HMD assumes a mediatory, communicative role in the society, facilitating the therapeutic and or healing process through social communication for problem solving that originates in the discipline of design. One way to actualize design is to have a shared metaphor and understand the others' feeling [62].

In the study, most of the studies in health communication have focused on the development of quality messages reflecting evidence about health behavior [63]. Communication in healthcare should have explicit aims, and at the same time, HMD should be actualized in the process of planning and developing interventions according to diverse populations or various situations. To carefully construct messages and adequately expose the messages, the underlying conceptual frameworks and models should be posed. The convergence approach based on philosophical and theoretical perspectives can give a direction for future research. However, because in this study only the theoretical phase of the conceptual framework was discussed, the remaining phases such as the fieldwork phase and the final analytical phase should be further studied.

Considering that HMD theoretically falls within the scope of the health information context where it exists in the form of meaning, rhythmicity, and co-transcendence, future research should be conducted to propose theoretically adequate constructs, to empirically test and validate the constructs, and examine the relationships between the constructs to generate empirical evidence [64]. The individual effects model, which focuses on individuals as they improve their knowledge and attitudes, and the social diffusion model, which leads to behavior change among social groups, may be considered to pose theoretical constructs within the context [63].

Previous research has consistently reported that a directional gap exists when conceived of communication. A majority of the studies show communications *from* providers *to* consumers, and the remainder show communications *between* providers and consumers [60]. Therefore, communications *from* consumers (i.e., self-reporting), *between* consumers (i.e., self-help groups), or *to* providers from another source (i.e., communication training) should be carefully designed at both the policy and programmatic levels [60, 63]. No matter how knowledgeable healthcare providers might be, if they are not able to successfully communicate with their consumers, they may not be of help.

Acknowledgements

The initial work of this study was presented at the International Association of Societies of Design Research 2015, Brisbane, Australia. The travel was fully supported by the National Research Foundation (NRF) of Korea Grant (NRF-2014S1A5B8044097) funded by the Korean Government, Korea. To further define and utilize social communication in healthcare, this study has been continuously developed by the support of Provost's Grant for Multidisciplinary Research (2018–2019) funded by Rutgers, The State University of New Jersey—Camden, USA, as well as the NRF of Korea Grant (NRF-2017S1A5B8066096).

Conflict of interest

The authors certify that there is no conflict of interest with any financial or non-financial interest in the subject matter or materials discussed in this manuscript.

Author details

Ji-Young An[1] and Jinkyung Paik[2*]

*Address all correspondence to: dejpaik@inje.ac.kr

1 School of Nursing, Rutgers, The State University of New Jersey, Camden, NJ, USA

2 Integrated u-Healthcare Design, Design Institute, College of Design, Inje University, South Korea

References

[1]   Oxford Dictionaries. [cited at 2017 Nov 5]. Available from: http://oxforddictionaries. com/us/definition/american_english/health?q=health

[2]   World Health Organization. Geneva. [cited at 2017 Oct 20]. Available from: http://www. who.int/about/en/

[3]   Center on Salutogenesis. The resource center on Salutogenesis at the University West. Sweden: [cited at 2017 Oct 29]. Available from: http://www.salutogenesis.hv.se/eng/ Related_concepts.8.html

[4]   Oxford Dictionaries. [cited at 2017 Nov 5]. Available from: http://oxforddictionaries. com/us/definition/american_english/healthcare?q=healthcare

[5]   White E. Public healthcare settings and health promotion. Healing HealthCare Systems; 2006: 1-29: [cited at 2018 January 20]. Available from: http://www.healinghealth.com/ images/uploads/files/SettingsPromoteHealth.pdf

[6]   An JY, Park TJ, Lee TK, Paik JK, Sung YJ. The publicness of healthcare design to enhance commodity values. Journal of Digital Interaction Design. 2012;**18**:173-186

[7]   Irving P, Dickson D. Empathy: Towards a conceptual framework for health profession-als. International Journal of Health Care Quality Assurance. 2004;**17**(4):212-220

[8]   Pfeil U, Zaphiris P. Patterns of Empathy in Online Communication. Proceedings of the SIGCHI Conference on Human Factors in Computing Systems. ACM. 2007. Available from: http://nguyendangbinh.org/Proceedings/CHI/2007/docs/p919.pdf

[9]   The Center for Health Design. [cited at 2018 April 18]. Available from: https://www. healthdesign.org/topics/communicationabout

[10] Sung YJ, An JY, Park TJ, Lee TK, Paik JK. Integrated u-healthcare design from the per-spective of medical humanities. Journal of The Korea Society of Health Informatics and Statics. 2012;**37**(1):12-21

[11] National Science Foundation. [cited at 2018 Feb 5]. Available from: https://www.nsf.gov/ od/oia/convergence/index.jsp

[12] Ulrich RS. Effects of interior design on wellness: Theory and recent scientific research. Journal of Health Care Interior Design. 1991;**3**:97-109

[13] Sung YJ, An JY, Paik JK. A review of concepts, characteristics, and guidelines of sup-portive design for healing environment. Archives of Design Research. 2013;**26**(1):507-523

[14] Wanzer MB, Booth-Butterfield M, Gruber K. Perceptions of health care providers' com-munication: Relationships between patient-centered communication and satisfaction. Health Communication. 2004;**16**(3):363-384

[15] Institute of Medicine. Washington, D.C.: National Academies Press; 2003

[16] Stewart MA. Effective physician-patient communication and health outcomes: A review. Canadian Medical Association Journal. 1995;**152**:1423-1433

[17] Stewart M, Brown J, Donner A, et al. The impact of patient-centered care on outcomes. The Journal of Family Practice. 1986;**49**:805-807

[18] Kim HS, editor. The Nature of Theoretical Thinking in Nursing. New York: Springer Publishing Company; 2000

[19] Schwartz-Barcott D, Kim HS. An expansion and elaboration of the hybrid model for concept development. In: Rodgers BL, Knafl KA, editors. Concept Development in Nursing: Foundations, Techniques and Applications. Philadelphia: W. B. Saunders; 1993. pp. 107-133

[20] Parse RR. Parse's human becoming. In: Parker ME, editor. Patterns of Nursing Theories in Practice. New York: National League for Nursing Press; 1993

[21] Oxford Dictionaries. [cited at 2017 Nov 5]. Available from: http://oxforddictionaries. com/us/definition/american_english/communication?q=communication

[22] Kant I. Critique of Judgement. (Pluhar WS, Trans.) Indiana, IN: Hackett publishing company, Inc.; 1984. (Original work published 1790)

[23] Kant I. Kant's Philosophy of History. (Lee HG, Trans.) Paju: Seogwangsa; 2009

[24] Fox FE, Rodham KJ, Harris MF, Taylor GJ, Sutton J, Scott J, Robinson B. Experiencing "the other side": A study of empathy and empowerment in general practitioners who have been patient. Qualitative Health Research. 2009;**19**(11):1580-1588

[25] Campbell RG, Babrow AS. The role of empathy in responses to persuasive risk communication: Overcoming resistance to HIV prevention messages. Journal of Health Communication. 2004;**16**(2):159-182

[26] Levinas E, Hand S, editors. The Levinas Reader. Oxford: Basil Blackwell; 1989 [cited at 2012 Mar 18]. Available from: http://noahbickart.fastmail.fm/TAL7175/Emmanuel%20 Levinas%20-%20The%20Levinas%20Reader.pdf

[27] Cassell EJ. The Nature of Suffering. Oxford: Oxford University Press; 2003

[28] Fostering artistic nursing potential through communication. Proceeding of the 2nd Eulji International Nursing Conference; 2012. October 11-12. [cited at 2012 Oct 30]. Available from: http://einc2012.topmeeting.org/

[29] Rogers CR. The necessary and sufficient conditions of therapeutic personality change. Journal of Consulting Psychology. 1957;**21**(2):95

[30] Schrooten I, de Jong M. If you could read my mind: The role of healthcare providers' empathic and communicative competencies in clients' satisfaction with consultations. Health Communication. 2017;**32**(1):111-118. DOI: 10.1080/10410236.2015.1110002

[31] Nightingale F. Notes on Nursing. New York: D. Broadway; Appleton and Company; 1860

[32] Santo LD, Pohl S, Saiani L, Battistelli A. Empathy in the emotional interactions with patients. Is it positive for nurses too? Journal of Nursing Education and Practice. 2014;**4**(2):74-81

[33] Branch WT. Teaching the human dimension of care in clinical settings. JAMA. 2001;**286**:1067-1074 PMid:11559292. http://dx.doi.org/10.1001/jama.286.9.1067

[34] Aring CD. Sympathy and empathy. Journal of the American Medical Association. 1958;**167**:448-452 http://dx.doi.org/10.1001/jama.1958.02990210034008

[35] Preston SD, de Waal FBM. Empathy: It's ultimate and proximate bases. The Behavioral and Brain Sciences. 2002;**25**:1-20

[36] Wispé L. Altruism, Sympathy, and Helping: Psychological and Sociological Principles. New York: Academic Press; 1978

[37] Sayumporn W, Gallagher S, Brown P, Evans J, Flynn V, Lopez V. The perception of nurses in their management of patients experiencing anxiety. Journal of Nursing Education and Practice. 2012;**2**(3):25-45 http://dx.doi.org/10.5430/jnep.v2n3p38

[38] Veloski J, Hojat M. Measuring Specific Elements of Professionalism: Empathy, Teamwork and Lifelong Learning. Oxford: Oxford University Press; 2006

[39] Johnson M. The Body in the Mind: The Bodily Basis of Meaning, Imagination, and Reason. Chicago: University of Chicago Press; 1987

[40] Parrot R. Emphasizing "communication" in health communication. Journal of Health Communication. 2004;**54**(4):751-761

[41] Oxford Dictionaries. [cited at 2017 Nov 5]. Available from: http://oxforddictionaries.com/us/definition/american_english/design?q=design

[42] Kim MS. A Cultural Navigation on the 21st Century's Design: Dialectics of Design, Culture and Symbol. Seoul: Sol Press; 1998. pp. 4-11

[43] Papanek V. Design for the Real World: Human Ecology and Social Change. Seoul: Miejinsa; 1995: 15-16

[44] Jensen JD. Addressing health literacy in the design of health messages. In: Cho HY, editor. Health Communication Message Design. California: SAGE; 2012. pp. 171-190

[45] Teso G, Ceppi G, Furlanetto A, Dario C, Scannapieco G. Defining the role of service design in healthcare. Design Management Review. 2013;**24**:40-47. DOI: 10.1111/drev.10250

[46] Maher L, Hayward B, Hayward P, Walsh C. Increasing patient engagement in healthcare service design: A qualitative evaluation of a co-design programme in New Zealand. Patient Experience Journal. 2017;**4**(1):23-32

[47] Jethwani K, Ling E, Mohammed M, Myint-U K, Pelletier A, Kvedar JC. Diabetes connect: An evaluation of patient adoption and engagement in a web-based remote glucose monitoring program. Journal of Diabetes Science and Technology. 2012;**6**(6):1328-1336

[48] Agboola S, Havasy R, Myint- UK, Kvedar J, Jethwani K. The impact of using mobile-enabled devices on patient engagement in remote monitoring programs. Journal of Diabetes Science and Technology. 2013;**7**(3):623-629

[49] [cited at 2012 Oct 4]. Available from: http://www.interiordesign.net/article/483463-Northwestern_Health_Care_Facility_Wins_Vista_Award.php?intref=sr

[50] Martsolf DS, Mickley JR. The concept of spirituality in nursing theories: Differing world-views and extent of focus. Journal of Advanced Nursing. 1998;**27**(2):294-303

[51] McEwen M, Wills EM, editors. Theoretical Basis for Nursing. Philadelphia: Lippincott Williams & Wilkins; 2011

[52] Lee CS, Kim SJ, Kweon YR. Theory: Parse's human becoming theory in practice and research. Nursing Research. 2006;**14**(2):122-158

[53] Lee KO, Kim MJ. Parse's human becoming theory: Analysis and evaluation by kim's coherence model. Chonnam Journal of Medical Sciences. 1998;**3**(1):75-90

[54] Fawcett J. The nurse theorists: 21st-centuryupdates-rosemarierizzoparse. Nursing Science Quarterly. 2001;**14**(2):126-131

[55] Parse RR. Transforming research and practice with the human becoming theory. Nursing Science Quarterly. 1997;**10**(4):171-174

[56] Smith MC. Pattern in nursing practice. Nursing Science Quarterly. 2007;**3**(2):55-56

[57] Gilligan C. In a Different Voice: Psychological Theory and Women's Development. Cambridge: Harvard University Press; 1982

[58] Lee KA, Song YH, Jang HM. A study on development of convergence design educating concept model (CDECM) for specialized design education: Focusing on a case of a com-munication design department at Korea national university of transportation. Journal of Digital Interaction Design. 2012;**12**(3):201-210

[59] Kang NH. Artificial forest and poetic justice or social aesthetics and communes. Moonwhagwahak. 2008;**53**:23-50

[60] Hill S. Directions in health communication. Bulletin of the World Health Organization. 2009;**87**:648-648

[61] Carper BL. Fundamental patterns of knowing in nursing. Advances in Nursing Science. 1978;**1**(1):13-18

[62] Papanek V. Design for Human Scale. New York: Van Nostrand Reinhold; 1983

[63] Hornik RC. Public health communication: Making sense of controdictory evidence. In: Hornik RC, editor. Public Health Communication: Evidence for Behavior Change. New Jersey: Taylor & Francis; 2008. pp. 1-19

[64] Fawcell J. The Relationship of Theory and Research. Philadelphia: FA Davis Company; 1999

Social Marketing: Application in Global Health

Chapter 4

Social Marketing for Health: Theoretical and Conceptual Considerations

Mohsen Shams

Additional information is available at the end of the chapter

http://dx.doi.org/10.5772/intechopen.76509

Abstract

Marketing, besides education and enforcement, is a strategy to change behaviors. The most important question for commercial marketers is: "What can we do to persuade people to buy our products?" They try to use commercial marketing principles such as exchange theory, consumer orientation, competition, audience segmentation, and marketing mix, to influence customers and sell their products and services. Health is considered as an important market, and people have to pay tangible and intangible costs to buy health products, services, and behaviors. So, health professionals must know about marketing key concepts and designing programs to promote health products and changing health behavior. "Social marketing" is an approach to persuade people to accept ideas and attitudes, perform healthy behaviors, refer to health facilities, and receive health products. In this chapter, the theoretical considerations and practical steps for planning, implementing, and evaluating the interventions based on the social marketing approach will be discussed. At the end of the chapter, we will study four researches designed and implemented based on the social marketing model.

Keywords: social marketing, health behaviors, behavior change

1. Introduction

More than 60 years ago, Wiebe asked a revolutionary question: "Why can't you sell brotherhood like soap?" He compared the principles and techniques for selling a tangible commercial product (soap) and promoting an intangible social idea (brotherhood) and concluded that key perspectives, principles, and tactics adapted from commercial marketing can be used in social behavior change [1]. In 1971, *social marketing* was born, when Kotler and Zaltman published their leading paper in Journal of Marketing and realized that the same marketing principles

IntechOpen

that were being used to sell products to customers could be used to "sell" ideas, attitudes, and behaviors [2]. Andreasen's defined social marketing as: "The application of commercial marketing technologies to the analysis, planning, execution and evaluation of programs designed to influence the voluntary behavior of target audiences in order to improve their personal welfare and that of their society" [3]. Rothschild believed that social marketing employs the principles of commercial marketing to influence consumer behavior and decision-making and attempts to influence voluntary behavior by offering or reinforcing incentives and/or consequences in an environment that invites voluntary exchange [4]. The Centers for Disease Control and Prevention (CDC) has introduced health marketing as an innovative approach that draws from traditional marketing theories and principles and adds science-based strategies to prevention, health promotion, and health protection. CDC defined health marketing as: "Creating, communicating, and delivering health information and interventions using customer-centered and science-based strategies to protect and promote the health of diverse populations" [5].

Healthcare providers supply products (e.g., iron or multivitamin supplements for infants, condoms for sex workers, and contraceptives for teenagers) and provide services (e.g., pap smear testing for early detection of cervical cancer, mammography for diagnosis of breast cancer, and chest X-ray for patients suspected with tuberculosis). But, that is not all. In healthcare systems, the people as consumers or clients are encouraged to perform healthy behaviors and avoid non-healthy behaviors. We ask them have enough physical activity, reduce their salt intake, consume enough fruit and vegetables, and quit smoking.

Health behavior is a behavior directed at promoting, protecting, and maintaining health, as well as reducing disease risks and early death. It includes personal attributes such as beliefs, expectations, values, perceptions, prevention, behavior patterns, actions, and habits that relate to health maintenance, restoration, and improvement [6]. In public health, education, marketing, and law enforcement are three main approaches applied to achieve behavior change. For people who consider the behavior change but do not have the required knowledge or skills, education is effective. Enforcement of laws and regulation is appropriate for the entrenched people who have no desire to change and resist deliberately. Marketing can be useful to bridge the gap between these two approaches and will be a good solution for those who are aware of the need to change but have not considered changing [7].

Health can be considered as a real market in which consumers pay the monetary and non-monetary costs and obtain the benefits of health products, services, or behaviors. If the marketing principles and techniques are applied, we can expect to be successful in selling our products, especially health behaviors. This chapter will address the theoretical concepts and practical steps for planning, implementing, and evaluating the interventions based on the social marketing approach for health.

2. Key concepts of social marketing

Health interventions to be considered as social marketing programs need to fulfill some criteria. The benchmark criteria provide a useful framework for assessing the extent to which an intervention is consistent with the social marketing approach and for identifying opportunities to potentially increase the impact of an intervention. Kotler and Lee explained some features of the social marketing approach: (1) focusing on understanding the perspectives of the full range of target audiences necessary to bring about change; (2) developing a research-based program, relying on formative research to develop and test concepts with members of the target audience; and (3) recognizing the need to include all elements of the marketing mix (i.e., product, price, place, promotion) to bring about behavior change [8]:

The National Social Marketing Centre has developed a set of eight social marketing benchmark criteria to promote the understanding and use of core social marketing concepts. They are behavior, customer orientation, theory, insight, exchange, competition, segmentation, and methods mix [9]. According to Andreasen's benchmark criteria [10], for an intervention to be classified as social marketing, at least one of the following components is needed. They are considered as the key concepts of the social marketing approach:

- Behavioral change: Determining the objective aiming to achieve behavioral change as the main focus of social marketing interventions.

- Formative research: Using audience research to understand target audiences, pre-test interventions and monitor their delivery; it is fundamental in social marketing interventions.

- Segmentation: Dividing a general target audience into smaller and homogenous segments based on the shared characteristics.

- Marketing mix: Adopted from the commercial sector is the marketing mix, also known as the 4Ps: product, price, place, and promotion [11]. These four key elements of social marketing are central to the planning and implementation of an integrated marketing strategy. Each of these four components should be present in a marketing plan. However, it is the science of correctly using these elements in combination with one another that provides the effective "marketing mix." To have an effective social marketing program, we must have a product developed based on the consumers' wants, needs, and preferences, priced realistically, distributed through convenient channels, and actively promoted to customers.

- Exchange: Social marketing programs aim to change behavior by establishing an exchange between the consumers and the program developer based on the consumers' wants and needs. In this exchange, consumers give up something of value and receive something of equal or greater value. Target audiences have opportunities to exchange their monetary and non-monetary resources for attractive tangible and/or intangible benefits. They are looking for the benefits of the product and have to pay its cost. Exchange forms voluntarily. Consumers want to fulfill their felt needs or desires and are ready to pay the costs and the social, economic, and physical costs (price). The costs must not be more than the perceived gains and benefits of the product.

- Competition: In a dynamic marketplace, commercial or social, there are different priorities and choices. So, competition is always present. If the target audience is not ready or willing to buy our promoted products, or we do not provide the products which the target audience wants, the marketing attempts will fail. In other words, the consumer will exit our market and go somewhere else. In case of social marketing, particular decisions are faced with some barriers that may result in highlighted desirability or perceived relative value of other options. So, thinking about competition is a major requirement in a successful social marketing program.

3. Planning of social marketing interventions

A health intervention defined as: "Any health-related measure taken to improve the health of an individual or a community; this may involve diagnosing, preventing, treating, and managing disease conditions, injury, or disability" [6]. In practice, understanding the key components of social marketing is not sufficient and we need to use social marketing planning models. Some of these models are the Social Marketing Assessment and Response Tool (SMART) model of Neiger & Thackeray (1998), Andreasen's model (1995), a framework suggested by Walsh, Rudd, Moeykens, and Moloney [15], and Weinreich's model (1999) [12]. All of them have practical phases and researchers can design the intervention step by step. The SMART model is a social marketing planning model developed by Neiger in 1998 and is applied to some researches in the health field [13, 14]. This model has seven phases as below:

3.1. Phase 1: Preliminary planning

Preliminary planning includes identification of the intended health problem, developing the goals, preparing the evaluation plan, and estimating the program costs. Like other programs, the first step is determining the health problems and selecting the prioritized ones. To get ready, behavioral aspects of the intended health problem were considered and the target health behavior was determined. According to this health behavior, we set the program goals. Evaluation planning, or determining measures of success, would include identifying and comparing measures before and after the intervention. Social marketers must estimate the monetary and non-monetary costs and try to provide them. Remember that social marketing programs are usually expensive interventions and advocacy with decision-makers is required.

3.2. Phases 2–4: Formative research

Formative research findings provide the primary idea for intervention. This data determines the target audience and its properties, the specific objectives, the primary idea for intervention, and communicating manners to the audience. Data are collected through qualitative approaches (focus group discussions (FGDs) and in-depth interviews) and quantitative surveys. After collecting and analyzing the formative research data, social marketers describe the target audience: who they are, what is important to them, what influences their behavior, and what would enable them to engage in the desired behavior. Formative research consists of audience, channels, and market analysis as below:

- Audience analysis: In this step, identification of the general target audience, segmentation, defining the special target segment, and then studying their needs, wants, and preferences were done. Learning about demographic, psychosocial, and behavioral variables through qualitative and quantitative methods is necessary for segmenting the primary general target audience into smaller and more homogenous subgroups and developing the particular interventions needed to modify risky behaviors. When we have a general and heterogeneous audience, their points of view about the target behavior, benefits, and barriers to perform behavior, and channels for communicating to the audience, are different. So, the segmentation of a general and large audience group to small and relatively homogeneous subgroups helps the planners to design an effective program. In this way, it is possible to develop marketing strategies customized to the unique characteristics of each subgroup and have better outcomes. We will discuss about segmentation later in formative research and market analysis. The target audiences were asked about the costs and benefits of performing the intended behavior, desires, and values. Qualitative and quantitative studies provide data for knowing the consumer's perspective before starting the strategy design. The data can be collected through surveys, focus groups, and in-depth interviews.

- Market analysis: For analyzing the market, the partners, the competitors, and the components of marketing mix are identified. Partners are those people or organizations who can help achieve the program goals. They have common, but not the same, goals and can provide the resources and support the activities. Competitors are those who provide similar products and services and may lose their benefits during our programs. So, they are vying for individual audience members' time and attention. Market analysis is not completed without marketing mix establishment. Marketing mix is also referred to as the 4Ps: product, price, place, and promotion. Product refers to the set of benefits associated with the desired behavior or service usage. To be successful, the product must provide a solution to problems that consumers consider important and must offer them a benefit they truly value. So, we need to research to understand people's wants, needs, and preferences. The marketing objective is to discover which benefits have the greatest appeal to the target audience and to design a product that provides those benefits. The product can be a tangible good or an intangible one. In the case of social marketing, behaviors are common products. The product can include ideas and behavior changes or something offered to the consumer to satisfy a want or need. Examples may include educational programs, screenings, environmental changes, self-care programs, and so on. Price refers to the cost for the promised benefits or the barriers that may prevent the consumer from taking action. This cost is always considered from the consumer's point of view. Costs can include money, time, opportunity, energy, social, behavioral, geographic, physical, structural, psychological factors, and convenience or pleasure. So, price is not always monetary and usually encompasses intangible costs. In setting the right price, it is important to know if consumers prefer to pay more to obtain "value-added" benefits and if they think that products given away or priced low are inferior to more expensive ones. Place: For tangible goods, place refers to the distribution system and the location of sales and for intangible products such as services or behaviors, it refers to the location where consumers can obtain information about the product. Promotion is often the most visible component of marketing. It includes the type of persuasive communication that marketers use to deliver the product benefits of tangible goods or intangible products and services. Promotional activities may encompass advertising, public relations, printed materials, promotional items, signage, special events and displays, face-to-face selling, and entertainment media [15]. For the exchange to take place, the social marketer must understand consumers' preferences regarding the 4Ps.

- Channel analysis: Identification of the best way to communicate to the target audience and know about their preferred sources of information is the main mission of channel analysis. Channels can be people, institutions, organizations, and specific communication techniques, such as mass media, personal communication, or public events. Social marketers may consider printed materials (e.g., pamphlet and brochures), printed media (e.g., newspapers and magazines), and mass media (e.g., radio and television programs, websites contents, social networks, and mobile applications).

3.3. Phase 5: Development

During the formative research, the main ideas for intervention are determined, and primary materials develop. Before completing the production of messages and materials for implementation, it is required to pretest the key elements including methods, communications, and strategies. They are presented to some members of the target audience and receive their feedback. Modifications are made based on the feedback. Typical methods for pretesting include focus groups, interviews, and surveys.

3.4. Phase 6: Implementation

Implementation is the activation of all strategies, tactics, and methods that were developed to achieve the designated goals and objectives. Activities such as the initiation of a mass-media awareness campaign, offerings of small-group self-management classes, or creation of a community coalition to improve the health behavior in a neighborhood are included in this phase.

3.5. Phase 7: Evaluation

Evaluation determines the program's success. It is done during and at the end of the intervention. When the quality of the program is assessed by documenting the extent to which it was implemented as designed, *process evaluation* has been done. In this type of evaluation, it is determined whether the program is operating as expected and whether there are areas in need of improvement. Consumer orientation, as a key concept of the social marketing process, means continually returning to the target audience and getting their reaction and point of view regarding the program. The number of self-management classes, radio programs or television advertising messages, pamphlets and brochures distributed, and posters installed in target audience neighborhoods can be the measures checked through process evaluation. The evaluation of the intervention effects, including impact evaluation and outcome evaluation, is very important in social marketing. Outcome measures could include changes in overall health status such as the mortality rate of cardiovascular diseases or prevalence rate of hypertension, while the impact measures would include improvements in health behaviors such as smoking and physical activity [16].

4. Application of social marketing in health programs

Gordon et al. [17] described three systematic reviews and primary studies that evaluate social marketing effectiveness. They concluded that social marketing provides a very promising framework for improving health both at the individual level and at the wider environmental and policy levels [17]. Morris and Clarkson [18] reviewed the studies using a social marketing framework for changing healthcare practice. They found social marketing as a useful solution-focused framework for systematically understanding barriers to individual behavior change and designing interventions accordingly. They argued that the social marketing approaches being adopted in public health may also provide a potent strategy for achieving change from practitioners and concluded that this approach provides a single framework to analyze and address the complex problem of behavior change, systematically using methods proven in commercial marketing [18]. Firestone et al. [19] reviewed the evidence of the effectiveness of social marketing in low- and middle-income countries, focusing on major areas of investment in global health: HIV, reproductive health, child survival, malaria, and tuberculosis. They concluded that social marketing can influence health behaviors and health outcomes in global health; however, evaluations assessing health outcomes remain comparatively limited. Evidence exists that social marketing can influence health behaviors and health outcomes [19]. Luca and Suggs [20] reviewed systematically 17 articles published after 1990. These articles reported social marketing interventions for the prevention or management of some diseases and behavioral risk factors, conducted evaluations, and met the six social marketing benchmarks' criteria. They concluded that there is an ongoing lack of use or underreporting of the use of theory in social marketing interventions and focused on applying and reporting theory to guide and evaluate interventions [20].

To obtain newer findings, we searched PubMed database using "social marketing "and found that 1655 articles have been published since 2010 till now. By limiting the search to "Systematic Reviews," 120 articles were determined, and by limiting the search more to behaviors, it showed that in 65 systematic review articles, social marketing interventions focused on behaviors. Application of social marketing to reduce tobacco use (19 articles) and alcohol consumption (18 articles), modify the nutritional practice (16 articles), promote physical activity (14 articles), and increase the condom usage (7 articles) were the most common subjects. Some particular systematic reviews in which "social marketing" has been mentioned in their titles are explained as below:

Xia et al. [21] reviewed 92 social marketing interventions published during 1997–2013. They concluded that if the six benchmarks of social marketing interventions (behavior change, consumer research, segmentation and targeting, exchange, competition, and marketing mix) are considered, and if the researchers analyze the audience, make the target behavior tangible, and promote the desired behavior, it is an effective approach in promoting physical activity among adults [21]. In another systematic review done by Luecking et al. [22], they searched PubMed, ISI Web of Science, PsycInfo, and the Cumulative Index of Nursing and Allied Health systematically to identify interventions targeting nutrition and/or physical activity behaviors of children enrolled in early care centers between 1994 and 2016. They concluded that social marketing could be an important strategy for preventing early childhood obesity through promoting physical activity and nutrition modification [22].

Aceves-Martins et al. [23] reviewed 38 non-randomized and randomized controlled trials conducted from 1990 to April 2014 in participants aged 5–17. They searched the PubMed, Cochrane, and ERIC databases to find the studies that contained social marketing strategies to reduce youth obesity in European school-based interventions. They concluded that the inclusion of at least five social marketing benchmark criteria in school-based interventions could be effective to prevent obesity in young people [23].

Sweat et al. [24] searched the National Library of Medicine's Gateway (includes Medline and AIDSline), PsycINFO, Sociological Abstracts, CINAHL, and EMBASE to study the effectiveness of social marketing for promoting condom use. Their meta-analyses showed a positive and statistically significant effect on increasing condom use, and all individual studies showed positive trends. They concluded that the cumulative effect of condom social marketing over multiple years could be substantial [24].

Janssen et al. [25] reviewed six papers extracted through searching PubMed, PsychInfo, Cochrane, and Scopus to describe the effects of an alcohol prevention intervention developed according to one or more principles of social marketing. Based on this review, the effect of applying the principles of social marketing in alcohol prevention in changing alcohol-related attitudes or behavior could not be assessed [25].

Wei et al. [26] searched the following electronic databases for results from January 1, 1980 to the search date July 14, 2010: Cochrane Central Register of Controlled Trials (CENTRAL), EMBASE, LILACS (Latin America and Brazil), PsycINFO, PubMed, Web of Science/Web of Social Science, Chinese National Knowledge Infrastructure (CNKI), and CQ VIP (China). This review provided limited evidence that multi-media social marketing campaigns can promote HIV testing among men who have sex with men (MSM) in developed countries. Future evaluations of social marketing interventions for MSM should employ more rigorous study designs. Long-term impact evaluations (changes in HIV or STI incidence over time) are also needed. Implementation research, including detailed process evaluation, is needed to identify elements of social marketing interventions that are most effective in reaching the target population and changing behaviors [26].

5. Lessons we learned from social marketing studies

1. Social marketing is an approach to change health behaviors. It can provide a useful framework for systematically understanding barriers to and benefits of the targeted health products.

2. Social marketing programs are based on the six benchmark criteria: focusing on behavior change, consumer research, audience segmentation, exchange, competition thinking, and establishing the marketing mix or 4Ps. For applying social marketing in practice, we need some planning models that contain operational steps and constructs. The SMART model is one of these planning models.

3. Formative research is the heart of social marketing programs, and audience, market, and channel analysis are three fundamental components of formative research.

4. Using social marketing to promote health behaviors is growing, but answering this question that whether the social marketing framework provides an effective means of bringing about behavior change remains an empirical question which still has to be tested in practice. However, many lessons have been learned in recent years.

6. Application of social marketing in health: some case studies in Iran

6.1. Reducing risky driving behaviors among taxi drivers in Tehran, Iran

In Iran, the mortality rate due to road traffic crashes is considerably high, and risky driving behavior by road users is an important factor influencing this health problem. However, many attempts have been made to reduce risky driving behaviors; they have been limited to education and enforcement. In this study, researchers designed and implemented an intervention based on the SMART (Social Marketing Assessment and Response Tool) model to reduce two specific risky driving behaviors, tailgating and non-driving between lines, among taxi drivers in Tehran, Iran. The target audience were the professional drivers in two municipality regions with the highest rate of traffic violations as recorded by the Tehran Driving Police. Formative research inclusive of a qualitative study and a quantitative survey was designed and implemented to determine intervention components. In a qualitative study, opinions and views of 42 taxi drivers in 4 focus group discussions were explored. They talked about the current driving in Tehran, causes of risky driving behaviors, suggested practices for modification of risky driving behaviors, appropriate places for introducing products and services, and appropriate channels to communicate and influence taxi drivers. Taxi drivers believed that if they concentrate on driving, they can avoid risky driving behaviors. Most of them suggested reminding messages for drivers and using materials containing these messages. Getting help from taxi route supervisors was suggested by taxi drivers as influencing people and effective communication channels.

Based on the formative research, the social marketing-based intervention was designed. The product was the reminder message for concentrating on the avoidance of two target behaviors, and the messages containing stickers were developed and installed on the glass before the driver's eyes. In addition, developing and distributing the message containing pamphlets, and justifying taxi route supervisors as opinion leaders to communicate messages to taxi drivers, were done. After 6 weeks, two target risky driving behaviors were assessed by checklists and compared.

Before the intervention, 68.3% of drivers in the intervention group and 77.1% of drivers in the control group committed tailgating, while after the intervention, these percentages were 36.9 and 67.9% in intervention and control groups respectively. For non-driving between lines, it was similar. Before the intervention, 60.9% of drivers in the intervention group and 59.0% of drivers in the control group committed non-driving between lines, while after the intervention, these percentages were 38.9 and 52.4%, respectively. The interventions resulted in statistically significant reductions in the two target behaviors in the intervention group as compared with the control group. Furthermore, logistic regression showed that the odds ratio for avoiding tailgating and non-driving between lines increased significantly in the intervention group: 2.34 (1.30–4.21) and 1.83 (1.06–3.17), respectively [27].

6.2. Using personal protective equipment (PPE) in workplaces

Workplace injury is the second leading cause of fatal injuries in Iran. However, many programs have been implemented to reduce workplace injuries; a majority of the interventions had been designed based on viewpoints of health and industry experts and were not consumer orientated. These interventions were usually focused on education and enforcement. In other words, for people who face a choice with attractive alternatives, or barriers, a third approach is needed; there was not any solution. In this study, an intervention based on the SMART model was designed and implemented to persuade workers in two constructing subway stations to use personal protective equipment (PPE) at the workplaces in Isfahan, Iran. This study is a quasi-experimental intervention based on the SMART model. A total of 44 employees in two separate subway stations under construction in Isfahan were assigned into intervention and control groups. All constructing subway stations were listed and one of them was selected as an intervention station randomly. By considering the similarities in the number and composition of employees in all stations, another one was considered as the control station. Intervention and control stations were in the north and center regions of Isfahan, respectively. Formative research included a qualitative study and a quantitative survey was designed. In the qualitative study, focus group discussions (FGDs) were used to explore viewpoints of the audience about PPE usage. The participants were asked to talk about the importance of using PPE, factors that influence their use and strategies to increase the use of PPE. In the quantitative study, attitudes and self-reported behaviors were measured by a 28-item questionnaire. Workers in both intervention and control stations completed the questionnaires and a 10-item checklist was used by two trained observers to record observed behaviors regarding PPE use. Based on initial findings, a free package containing a well-designed light-weighted helmet, a dust mask and safety gloves were delivered to workers in the intervention group. A sticker with an emotionally tailored message reminding them of the importance of caring for themselves because of their families was attached to the helmet. This message was developed based on concerns expressed by the workers during FGDs. They had told that their families were the most important reason for using PPE because injuries would result in problems not only for themselves but also for their families. Providing and delivering a free and suitable package containing PPE in the workplace and promoting the product through personal communication and applying printed materials were its main components. The intervention was done in the workplace, and stickers with the message "I take care of myself because of my family" were attached to all helmets. In the package, we also put a simple tailored pamphlet including messages related to the advantages of using PPE and the risks they can reduce. For people who were unschooled, face-to-face counseling was held. The intervention was implemented for 4 weeks in the intervention station. Engineers and foremen supervised the use of PPE and reminded and warned the employees to use the package content. After 6 weeks, the use of PPE in both intervention and control stations were checked by checklists. Behaviors in the intervention and control stations were measured using an observational checklist. After the intervention, the percentage of workers who used PPE at the intervention station increased significantly. Before the intervention, none of the workers in intervention station used helmet and safety masks, and 4 and 12% of them in the control station used these PPEs. After the intervention, 43.5% of the intervention group and 27.3% of the control group used helmets, and 39.1% of the intervention group and 18.2% of the control group used safety masks and these percentages were 36.9 and 67.9% in intervention and control groups respectively. The intervention resulted in statistically significant reductions in the two target behaviors in the intervention group as compared with the control group [28].

6.3. Promoting mammography in Iranian women

Mammography has an important role in early detection of breast cancer. So, the health sector tries to persuade women to do that. A majority of the interventions are based on education and information and there has been less attention to making mammography cost beneficent. This study aimed at assessing the effect of a social marketing-based intervention to persuade one to do mammography in Bojnord, Iran. In this study, two villages which had similar demographic characteristics such as population, sex ration, and socioeconomic status, considered as intervention and comparison groups randomly. All women of 35 years and older consisted of 343 women (151 in intervention and 191 in comparison groups) and were included in the study. To obtain the main idea for intervention, and exploring the viewpoints of the target group about mammography, a formative research combined of a quantitative survey and a qualitative study was done. It was completed by the women to assess their attitudes, and four focus group discussions were established to gather qualitative data. The quantitative study showed that time for referring and waiting in hospitals, financial costs, forgetting mammography, and fear of exposure to x-ray are more prominent. In the qualitative study, expending time and high economical costs are considered as two main factors related to not taking up mammography. According to the formative research findings, an intervention focused on the main barriers that were designed. Women who chose mammography were registered in health houses. After arranging the appointments with the local hospital, women were picked up in groups and brought to the hospital. A person who was familiar with the process of mammography welcomed them and coordinated the service. Mammography was not free, but a significant discount had been considered by the hospital. This program was implemented for 4 consecutive weeks. One week after the intervention, the number of mammograms in two villages was determined and compared. After the intervention, 48.1% of the women in the intervention group went for mammography and there were no changes in the comparison group [29].

6.4. Promoting normal vaginal delivery

The rate of Cesarean sections in Iran is higher than the acceptable rate recommended by the World Health Organization. Regardless of implementing many educational programs to reduce Cesarean section rates, some barriers are influencing the choices of pregnant women. This field trial was done in Yasuj, Iran, and 39 3–4 months pregnant primigravida were included in the study as the target audience. They chose Cesarean section for delivery. A formative research combined of a quantitative survey and a qualitative study was done to achieve the social marketing mix, and based on the results a tailored intervention was designed and pretested on the subjects. The product was a promoting package that consisted of a short-time instruction, messages for brief interventions in public health facilities, and a phone counseling service managed by trained midwives. The final intervention was implemented for a period of 1 month and its effectiveness was assessed after at least 1 month by a proportion test. One month after the intervention 30 pregnant women expressed willingness and intentions to have a normal delivery, which was a statistically significant change [30].

7. Conclusion

Education, marketing, and law enforcement are three key solutions for changing behaviors. For people who consider the behavior change but do not have the required knowledge or skills, education is effective. Enforcement of laws and regulation is appropriate for the entrenched people who have no desire to change and resist deliberately. Marketing can be useful to bridge the gap between these two approaches and will be a good solution for those who are aware of the need to change but have not considered changing. Healthcare system supplies the health products (e.g., iron or multivitamin supplements for infants, condoms for sex workers, and contraceptives for women who want to do family planning), provides the health services (e.g., pap smear testing for early detection of cervical cancer in women, mammography for early detection of breast cancer, and chest X-ray for patients suspected with tuberculosis), and encourages people to perform the right health behaviors (e.g., having enough physical activity, smoking cessation, and reducing salt intake). So, healthcare providers have something to offer their consumers and expect the audiences to take them. Health is an important social market in which the principles and key elements of commercial marketing are applied. To be successful in the health market, it is required to consider the key principles and techniques of social marketing such as consumer research, audience segmentation, exchange theory, competition thinking, and marketing mix by decision-makers, managers, and care providers. So, the future policy must be focused on empowering them to apply this approach as an important solution for health issues.

Although, attention to using the social marketing for health problems is expanding, there are some controversies about the long-term of the social marketing based programs yet. We need to conduct more and more trials to be sure. If the decision-makers in health systems want to solve their problems, they have to pay attention to social marketing as a new and innovative choice.

Conflict of interest

The author does not have any conflict of interest.

Author details

Mohsen Shams

Address all correspondence to: moshaisf@yahoo.com

School of Health, Yasuj University of Medical Sciences, Yasuj, Iran

References

[1] Wiebe GD. Merchandising commodities and citizenship on television. Public Opinion Quarterly. 1951;**15**(4):679-691. DOI: 10.1086/266353

[2] Kotler P, Zaltman G. Social marketing: An approach to planned social change. Journal of Marketing. 1971;**35**(3):3-12

[3] Andreasen AR. Social marketing: Its definition and domain. Journal of Public Policy and Marketing. 1994;**13**(1):108-114

[4] Rothschild ML. Carrots, sticks, and promises. A conceptual framework for the management of public health and social issue behaviors. Journal of Marketing. 1999;**63**:24-27

[5] Bernhardt JM. Improving health through health marketing. Preventing Chronic Disease. 2006;**3**(3):A73

[6] Modeste N, Tamayose T. Dictionary of Public Health Education and Promotion. 2004 San Francisco, CA: John Wiley & Sons, Inc. Jossey-Bass; 2004

[7] Maibach EW, Rothschild ML, Novelli WD. Social marketing. In: Glanz K, Rimer BK, Lewis FM. Health Behavior and Health Education. 3rd ed. San Francisco, CA: Jossey-Boss; 2002

[8] Lee N, Kotler P. Social Marketing: Changing Behaviors for Good. Sage Publications; 2015

[9] National Social Marketing Centre. NSMC benchmark criteria. 2010. Available from: http://www.socialmarketing-toolbox.com/content/nsmc-benchmark-criteria-0 [Accessed: 2018-01-30]

[10] Andreasen AR. Marketing social marketing in the social change marketplace. Journal of Public Policy and Marketing. 2002;**21**:3-13

[11] Kotler P, Roberto N, Lee N. Social Marketing: Improving the Quality of Life. 2nd ed. Thousand Oaks, CA: Sage; 2002

[12] Neiger BL, Thackeray RB, Barnes MD, McKenzie JF. Positioning social marketing as a planning process for health education. American Journal of Health Studies. 2003;**18**:75-81

[13] Neiger BL, Thackeray R. Application of the SMART model in two successful social marketing projects. American Journal of Health Education. 2002;**33**:291-293

[14] Thackeray R, Neiger BL. Use of social marketing to develop culturally innovative diabetes interventions. Diabetes Spectrum. 2003;**16**:15-20

[15] Walsh DC, Rudd RE, Moeykens BA, Moloney TW. Social marketing for public health. Health Affairs (Millwood). 1993;**12**(2):104-119

[16] Grier S, Bryant CA. Social marketing in public health. Annual Review of Public Health. 2005;**26**:319-339

[17] Gordona R, McDermotta L, Steada M, Angus K. The effectiveness of social marketing interventions for health improvement: What's the evidence? Public Health. 2006;**120**:1133-1139

[18] Morris ZS, Clarkson PJ. Does social marketing provide a framework for changing healthcare practice? Health Policy. 2009;**91**:135-141

[19] Firestone R, Rowe CJ, Modi SN, Sievers D. The effectiveness of social marketing in global health: A systematic review. Health Policy and Planning. 2017;**32**:110-124

[20] Luca NR, Suggs LS. Theory and model use in social marketing health interventions. Journal of Health Communication. 2013;**18**(1):20-40

[21] Xia Y, Deshpande S, Bonates T. Effectiveness of social marketing interventions to promote physical activity among adults: A systematic review. Journal of Physical Activity and Health. 2016;**13**(11):1263-1274

[22] Luecking CT, Hennink-Kaminski H, Ihekweazu C, Vaughn A, Mazzucca S, Ward DS. Social marketing approaches to nutrition and physical activity interventions in early care and education centers: A systematic review. Obesity Reviews. 2017;**18**(12):1425-1438

[23] Aceves-Martins M, Llauradó E, Tarro L, Moreno-García CF, Goretty T, Escobar T, et al. Effectiveness of social marketing strategies to reduce youth obesity in European school-based interventions: A systematic review and meta-analysis. Nutrition Reviews. 2016;**74**(5):337-351

[24] Sweat MD, Denison J, Kennedy C, Tedrow V, O'Reilly K. Effects of condom social marketing on condom use in developing countries: A systematic review and meta-analysis, 1990-2010. Bulletin of the World Health Organization. 2012;**90**(8):613-622A

[25] Janssen MM, Mathijssen JJ, van Bon-Martens MJ, van Oers HA, Garretsen HF. Effectiveness of alcohol prevention interventions based on the principles of social marketing: A systematic review. Substance Abuse Treatment, Prevention, and Policy 2013;**1**;8:18

[26] Wei C, Herrick A, Raymond HF, Anglemyer A, Gerbase A, Noar SM. Social marketing interventions to increase HIV/STI testing uptake among men who have sex with men and male-to-female transgender women. Cochrane Database Systematic Reviews. 2011;**7**(9):CD009337

[27] Majdzadeh R, Rashidian A, Shams M, Shojaeezadeh D, Montazeri A. Using the social marketing model to reduce risky driving behaviors among taxi drivers in Tehran. Scientific Journal of School of Public Health and Institute of Public Health Research. 2011;**9**(2):21-40

[28] Shamsi M, Pariani A, Shams M, Soleymani-nejad M. Persuasion to use personal protective equipment in constructing subway stations: Application of social marketing. Injury Prevention. 2016;**22**:149-152

[29] Shamsi M, Neyestani H, Ebrahimipour H, Esmaeili H, Vafaei Najjar A, Nosrati M. Using social marketing model to persuade the women to do mammography. Scientific Journal of School of Public Health and Institute of Public Health Research. 2014;**12**(1):85-96

[30] Maleki M, Mousavizadeh A, Parhizkar S, Shams M. Promotion of normal vaginal delivery among Primigravidae: An application of social Marketing in the Field of health. Scientific Journal of School of Public Health and Institute of Public Health Research. 2017;**14**(2):110-120

Social Marketing and Health Communication: A Case Study at the Brazilian Federal Senate

Paulo Ricardo dos Santos Meira, Ilana Trombka and
Daniele Carvalho Calvano Mendes

Additional information is available at the end of the chapter

http://dx.doi.org/10.5772/intechopen.78126

Abstract

This chapter aims to show how a breast cancer campaign can be successfully planned and how the expected results can be achieved, in accordance with the best practices of health communication under the social marketing paradigm. The case study is the Pink October (month dedicated to women's health) at the Brazilian Federal Senate, in 2017, result of interdepartmental (Top Management, Health, Human Resources and Social Communication areas) and interinstitutional (Federal Senate, Government of the Federal District and health-related institutions) partnership efforts. Social marketing, internal marketing and *endobranding* concepts are explored, as well as the breast cancer issue, in order to provide a better understanding among interested readers. While results are positive, some challenges and concerns are brought to light, which point to the need for improvements in the Pink October program for the coming years. The case study involved literature review, analysis of media articles and focused interviews.

Keywords: Brazil, breast cancer, Federal Senate, health communication, social marketing

1. Introduction

It is well known that in every society, the behavior of some individuals is not in line with the long-term interests of society as a whole [1]. Examples range from the lack of contraceptive use in countries with overpopulation, excessive production of hazardous waste and even careless driving. In this context, the importance of social marketing arises, and it can be defined as the use of marketing tools to promote planned social change [2]. However, the assessment of effectiveness of social marketing programs still presents a great challenge [3, 4]. This chapter aims to help readers understand some of the dimensions that can be used to assess the effectiveness of a given health program—in this case, the Pink October at the Brazilian Federal Senate. Additionally, although there is literature to corroborate the idea of social marketing as the use of marketing theory, skills and practices to achieve social change, especially through the use of online social media, we believe this should be treated simply as marketing on social media. We focus on this at the end of this chapter, with a practical approach on how this concept is used by the Brazilian legislative house. To start with, we shall go over the main concepts of social marketing and its internal use in institutions, especially regarding the employees and their families.

The case study involved literature review, analysis of internal and external media articles and focused interviews with the organizers and partners to create a short overview of the initiative and its future potential improvements.

2. Social marketing and health communication on breast cancer prevention in a public institution

This section aims to discuss the present status of breast cancer cases in Brazil, the basic definition of social marketing and its relation to health communication, as well as the field's best practices. Another main goal here is to bring up a discussion on internal marketing as a powerful tool to achieve an effective health communication, which may influence behaviors and attitudes toward other potential health issues, and finally, to present the Pink October case in detail.

2.1. Breast cancer

According to the Brazilian Ministry of Health, breast cancer is the type of cancer that mostly affects women countrywide, accounting for about 25% of the new cases each year. It is the second leading cause of cancer-related death in developed countries, falling only behind lung cancer [5]. The National Cancer Institute (Inca) reported that there are about 60,000 new breast cancer cases per year in Brazil, of which 15,000 lead to death.

According to the gynecologist Doctor Daniele Carvalho Mendes, the causes of the disease are varied, ranging from genetic mutations that might occur during a person's own lifetime up to certain changes to genes that control the way our cells function, especially how they grow and divide. Also, it can be caused by the habits that are proper of a social and/or cultural environment. Examples of such causes include alcohol abuse, overweight and a sedentary lifestyle. Doctor Mendes points out that clinical examination of the breasts should be performed annually by a gynecologist for women from the age of 25. Mammography should be done periodically after the woman reaches 40 years old. When necessary, the doctor may refer the patient to a mastologist for detailed examinations. As Doctor Mendes sees it, the possibility of having cancer is not cause for panic, since the treatment evolved to be increasingly individualized and based on the genetic profile of the tumor.

2.2. Understanding social marketing, internal marketing and branding

For a better understanding of the term endobranding or internal branding, it is important to conduct a brief review of the internal marketing and branding concepts in order to see that branding, in this case, can be both a marketing tool—the so-called "internal branding"—and also an applicable tool in the internal communication of social marketing campaigns [7, 37, 38]. It is worthwhile, as well, to go through the definition of social marketing and how it is connected to the two previous concepts.

2.2.1. Social marketing

A well-established definition of social marketing, is "[…] the use of marketing principles and techniques to influence a target audience to voluntarily accept, reject, modify or abandon a behavior for the benefit of individuals, groups or society as a whole" [8]. For Wilkie and Moore, social marketing originally developed itself as an area that would focus on "the work of nonprofitable groups and government agencies that dealt with effective intervention in areas of social problems," especially in public health programs as seen in Ling, Franklin, Lindsteadt and Gearon [9, 10].

This perspective of social marketing as a tool to encourage planned social change has been successfully used in different programs [11]. Nevertheless, although social marketing aimed at greater social welfare, the agents of such social change (governments, institutions, public policy makers) face complex ethical challenges [12, 13]. For Brenkert, the point goes beyond the moral issues faced by other forms of marketing such as accusations of manipulation and dishonesty and issues of intrusiveness [14].

The implementation of social marketing initiatives implies several challenges, as seen by Kotler and Lee, such as asking citizens to give up a pleasure (such as having to bathe more quickly), to be in a situation of eventual discomfort (such as wearing a seatbelt on buses and cars), resisting peer pressure (not starting to smoke), embarrassing situations (prostate examination), coping with sensitive situations (testing for AIDS),—challenges that may be added to asking citizens to reflect on issues that, at first, are difficult to grasp of are far from their immediate reality, such as the conservation of the oceans, among many others [15, 16]. For example, Peters et al. have demonstrated the low effectiveness of private sector initiatives in sexual and reproductive health campaigns in emerging countries for a number of difficulties [17]. Concerning health communication itself, Haider also enumerates several difficulties to face, for instance, the evaluation issue [18].

Hastings advocates that social marketing can take advantage of both external relationships among the stakeholders, and internal relationships such as the "domestic partnerships" of employees and functional departments of the organization [19]. In this context, we would have something that could be called a "social endomarketing" that could benefit from generic branding strategies, as referenced earlier. As the saying goes, "There is no better means of promoting another person's change of heart than allowing our own heart to be changed." (C. Terry Warner) [20]. In social marketing, that assumption remains true.

2.2.2. Internal marketing

The internal audience of an institution is important, be it as the selected target audience of a given social marketing campaign, or as a sample of a pre-stage testing for external campaigns. In the first case, one can use branding strategies, as advocated by Evans and Hastings in 2008, in the book "Public Health Branding: Applying Marketing for Social Change," a book that emphasizes the benefits of using branding strategies to social marketing, confirming what had been said by Keller in 1998 and consolidated in the work edited by Evans [21–23].

According to Gronroos, internal marketing is "a philosophy to manage the staff and a systematic way for developing and performing a service culture," a definition that moves into the quality of the service provided by the employees [24]. Nevertheless, we can see a broader approach in newer practices, social marketing included. Thus, just as there is B2B, business-to-business, and B2C, or business-to-consumer, we have the B2E, or business-to-employee, the marketing effort from the institution to its employees, as explained by Kotler and Keller. One example is the Disney Institute seminars on "Disney Style," intended for their own employees, but also for employees from other organizations around the world who participate in these meetings [25].

Kotler and Keller also clarify that internal marketing describes the process of training and motivating employees so that they meet the customers' needs. He states that "the greatest contribution that can be given by the marketing department is to be exceptionally skilled at inducing other parts of the organization to do marketing." In the words of Costa [26]:

> "The internal marketing and internal communication (although, in practice, they are often accepted as synonyms, internal communication is in fact part of the compound internal marketing) have a decisive role not only in the identification of this demand, but also in building the sense of belonging to the organization and satisfaction of the employees' desires. Besides the tangible attributes of the relationship between the organization and the employee, you also must to know how to communicate subjective values. Before satisfying the external public, the organization needs to meet its workforce."

Internal marketing aims to strengthen the internal relations of the organization with the mission of integrating the notions of customer and internal supplier; it intends to forge a shared view of the institution's business among the employees, including of themes such as management, goals, results, products, services and markets in which it operates, but it also seeks to "convince" employees of a given social cause, as seen in the example presented later in this chapter.

The view and the concept of internal marketing, in the strategic levels of the organization, are key points that are in the core of the process. An initial diagnosis, followed by an implementation plan that takes into account the reality of the company is another key factor to ensure the desired results of the process. Among other factors that should be considered are the visual impact of instruments and the most appropriate branding strategy for internal messages in order to guarantee their success.

2.2.3. Internal branding

Brand management, or branding, "is a basic decision in an organization where it uses a name, a slogan, a design, symbols or a combination of all these to identify its products or the institution itself," according to Kerin et al. [27].

It is also important to see that the organization's brand must be related to "people," to the way they attribute meaning to this brand, and this is a two-way street: it must focus on "endorsers," that is, people who will defend the brand in different situations, and to the "employees" who must also learn to connect the brand with the company and grasp their values and meaning from it [6].

Strategic brand management starts with decisions regarding a particular brand identity that the organization wishes to have toward the market (as it wants to be seen), and then goes to the management to ensure, as far as possible, that brand image (how it is in fact perceived) in accordance with the intended identity [9].

Carvajal also brings up this matter [28]:

> "All companies have the ability to radiate its own image, both outside and inside. Thus, we can think of an internal identity and external identity. The internal identity is generated into the organization and constitutes the cultural heritage (nonmonetary capital), or the corporate culture of a company, which is expressed in environmental values like order, cleanliness, good manners, goodwill at work, compliance with tasks and duties, etc. But there is a parallel external identity, i.e., the way in which ones' company is perceived by the outsider. It would be correct to conclude that the external and internal identity will depend on one another, and that the object of study of corporate image is the administration of all forms of identity."

When developing such inner identity, branding can play a very important role. Kotler and Keller define internal branding as the "activities and processes that help inform and inspire employees" [25]. As the branding per se is related to the management process of giving a brand to an idea or product, internal branding or endobranding is, for instance, the brand management of a social or motivational internal program. The brand helps in the understanding and it makes something tangible so it can be better perceived, understood and valued internally by employees of an organization.

Within the public sector, this need is also an issue. According to Dias [29]:

> "Motivated mainly by the movement of deploying strategic planning, the public sector has been developing an ever-closer look at some essential practices to achieve overall better results, and, consequently, on the internal communication and internal marketing strategy."

For Evans [23], the branding of social and health behaviors has become widespread and is now a central approach in social marketing. Thus, adequate branding, in social marketing programs, can enable a great deal of success, as it is also shown in Evans et al., when they examined a drug abuse campaign, which targeted young people. The same rationale could be used for internal campaigns, within organizations [30].

2.3. Social media: the new frontier for health communication

A report on the digital economy recently released (3) by the United Nations Conference on Trade and Development (UNCTAD) puts Brazil in fourth place in the world ranking of Internet users. With 120 million people connected, Brazil lags behind only the United States (242 million), India (333 million) and China (705 million). After Brazil, there are Japan (118 million), Russia (104 million), Nigeria (87 million), Germany (72 million), Mexico (72 million) and the United Kingdom (59 million) [31].

Regarding social media, their use in Brazil is also highlighted. More than 260 million people in Latin America, 42% of the total population, regularly access social networks. According to a survey by the eMarketer agency, 86.5% of users use smartphones to connect to networks. Brazil is the country with the most users of the continent, with a total of 93.2 million by the end of the 2017. In Mexico, there are 56 million, followed by Argentina with 21.7 million [32].

This growing expansion of social networks did not go unnoticed by the Brazilian Senate, which organized a seminar to better understand how different social networks have impacted both the politics itself and the logic of e-government and citizen participation [33]. Experts affirm that networks like Facebook, Twitter, YouTube and Instagram allow the public, which previously only received messages, to now produce content and intensify the impact that information and opinions can have, including regarding politics and the public image of institutions.

According to the Inter-Parliamentary Union (IPU)[1], as published in its guidelines for the use of social media by parliament members, "social networks" (also known as "Web 2.0") are a wide-ranging set of web-based tools that allow individuals to access, participate and interact with third parties (whether being individuals, companies or public-sector entities), when and how they wish [34].

2.4. The institutional social media of the Brazilian Senate

Social networks, or social media, have become systematically part of the Senate's everyday institutional life since 2010, initially as new media for the dissemination of facts and legislative news, but which evolved into interactivity with citizens and society in 2011 and have been increasingly used for corporate communication since 2013, with a more intensified work by the

---

[1]Founded in 1889, the IPU is the international organization that brings together representatives of parliaments of several sovereign states. Its purpose is to promote inter-parliamentary dialogue on a global level and work for peace and cooperation among peoples from the development of representative institutions [34]. The IPU was founded by William Randall Cremer and Frédéric Passy, who "envisioned an organization where conflicts were resolved through international arbitration." Thus, in order to mediate contacts between parliaments in a multilateral manner, the IPU acts preferentially in the following areas: "representative democracy, human rights and humanitarian law, gender equality, international trade, education, science and culture" ("União Interparlamentar," In: WIKIPEDIA PT, 2013).

Coordination of Advertising and Marketing. Since then, it has been an important tool to foster closer, more effective and efficient relationships between the Senate and different target audiences. This basically reinforces the line of action advocated by Schellong regarding the employment of CRM—Citizen Relationship Management systems—which bring technology, people and business processes together, and was conceived to be used by the public sector, as a business tool for developing closer ties between citizens and government institutions [35–38].

The Senate's profiles on the social media are divided basically into four categories: Institutional, Journalistic, Segmented and Public Service.

The institutional profiles (not journalistic or hard news, but institutional in nature) are as follows:

- Facebook: Senado Federal do Brasil

- Twitter: @senadofederal

- Google Plus: Senado Federal do Brasil

- Flickr: Você no Senado

- YouTube: SenadoBR

The information produced by the Senate has been reaching an increasingly higher number of people through social networks. In January 2016, the homepage on Facebook had 240,000 followers. In April 2017, it reached 1.7 million, a growth of almost 600% in the period.

The growth in the number of people reached by the messages is also high. In the same period, Facebook posts were shared 4.6 million times, received 15.5 million likes and generated 23.6 million comments. In recent months, the Senate's profile on Facebook has been the one with the world's largest engagement records among government websites, surpassing that of NASA and the White House, according to Quintly (www.quintly.com), a social media analysis site. The Quintly ranking considers the total number of followers of the Facebook profile and the number of people interacting with the posts, which is measured by the number of shares, likes and comments. The position in the ranking changes constantly, since it depends on the daily activity of the pages [54].

The Senate's social networks, as a whole, now have more than 3.5 million followers among Facebook, Twitter and Instagram, and are commonly referred to as benchmarks by other public institutions [39].

2.5. Social marketing programs of the Brazilian Senate

In 1997, the Senate created its Special Projects SubSecretariat—nowadays called Coordination of Advertising and Marketing—which was founded with the purpose of paying particular attention to promotional and institutional activities of the Senate. This new service, part of the Secretariat of Social Communication, would dedicate time and efforts to the institutional marketing of all areas of the Senate. With the mission of planning and developing internal and external campaigns, this sector was created to organize and take over dispersed tasks as well as the advertising creation of audiovisual products that were scattered throughout the legislative house [35]. In social media, advertising campaigns are disseminated primarily on institutional profiles in Facebook, Google Plus and Twitter networks. These campaigns can be divided into "institutional," "public utility" and "corporate," according to their main purpose. From 2015 on, the General Director of the Senate has gathered a small group of staff who responds directly to her in order to get a closer coordination of the internal communication initiatives, and that was the case of the Pink October 2017 edition.

3. Pink October case

Advances in coping with breast cancer and women's empowerment were the main focus of the Pink October campaign of 2017. The pink ribbon symbolizes the fight against the disease and the movement aims to stimulate the participation of the population, of businesses and of institutions and to warn women about prevention.

The Federal Senate has released the Pink October Campaign as part of its 2015 Commitment Letter, which arouse from the concern regarding the health and the quality of life of its servers, ratified by the 2017–2018 Strategic Objectives document, in which this concern is again mentioned, obtaining the full support of the institution. Since the Senate has the institutional motivation, the resources and the health statistics to corroborate the importance of this initiative, the project was thoroughly carried out by all the participants.

The release of the "Outubro Rosa" campaign against Breast Cancer was held on October 3, 2017, with the pink lighting act of the National Congress. The Procuradoria Especial da Mulher (Women's Special Attorneyship) and the Secretaria da Mulher da Câmara dos Deputados (Women's Secretariat of the House of Representatives), in partnership with the General Board and other sectors of the two Houses, came together once again to organize various events during the month.

In the 2017 program, significant actions were conducted, such as the special moment for the outsourced collaborators of the House who, in addition to taking part in the activities proposed for the day, obtained medical referral for a mammography examination with a professional follow-up.

There was also a close chat with mastologists, geneticists and gynecologists, during which the female staff were able to ask questions about breast cancer and other issues. The initiative was provided free of charge by a specialized institution [40].

According to Doctor Daniele Mendes, "everyone has a beloved wife, a sister, a mother, a friend, a co-worker." The main message today is to face the disease, knowing that medicine offers a wide range of effective treatments, especially for breast cancer. It is worth investing and insisting on the early diagnosis. She claims that campaigns such as the Pink October are important since, the more this relevant information is disseminated, the less fear will be faced by women when learning about a diagnosis. Knowledge is a powerful tool because it lowers the stigma that breast cancer is incurable. A well-informed woman can remain alert to her body and is more likely to discover an early-stage nodule with full healing possibilities [41].

3.1. Planning

An initial briefing took place in March 2017, in which the General Director of the Senate presented the initial ideas on the possibility of deepening and expanding the activities of the Pink October, traditionally carried out every year, aiming to extend the benefits to the outsourced employees of the Federal Senate. At the meeting, two mastologists from the Federal Senate, Doctor Daniele Carvalho Calvano Mendes and Doctor Martinho Cândido de Albuquerque dos Santos, constructively shared views and ideas consistent with the Director-General's initiative of deciding to offer breast cancer exams—mammograms—over the public health services network to outsourced employees. In order to achieve this goal, the Directors of the Senate contacted the Health Secretary of the Federal District Government and consolidated the partnership, without any direct costs for this economically disadvantaged public.

Contacts were also made with the Internal Communication team of the Social Communication Secretariat of the Senate, so that a wide dissemination network could be formed. In a technical meeting with the area, other Secretariat teams were convened, so that an internal communication effort could be made in order to have available all the communication means of the institution, such as social media, web portal, newspaper, TV and radio of the Federal Senate, whose scope is relevant in terms of reaching out to the public.

The Department of Quality of Life at Work has been assigned as well to collaborate in the process.

In the case of the Pink October, the brand development for such an endobranding initiative has been created by an art director who works for the General Director staff, Mr. Thomas Cortes, responsible for creating other internal campaigns as well. The brand shows the silhouette of the National Congress (Federal Senate + House of Representatives) inside a rose (**Figure 1**).

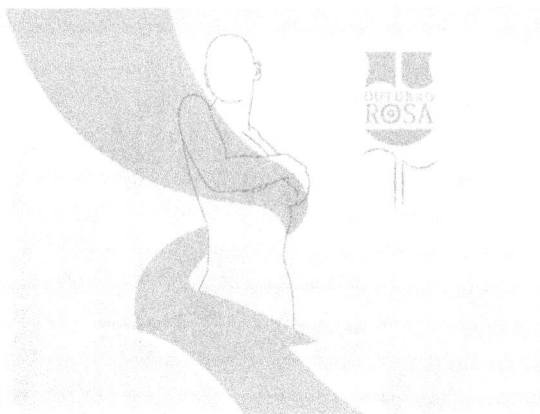

Figure 1. Pink October brand.

3.2. Execution

The release of the Pink October campaign on breast cancer occurred on the night of October 3, with the lighting act of the National Congress. The Procuradoria Especial da Mulher (Women's Special Attorneyship) and the Secretaria da Mulher da Câmara dos Deputados (Women's Secretariat of the House of Representatives), in partnership with other sectors of the two Houses, came together once again to organize various events during the month in order to warn society about the importance of prevention of this disease which is among the main causes of death amid women aged 30–69 (**Figure 2**).

On October 9, the outsourced collaborators started being forwarded to the place where the mammography exam would be conducted. This was an initiative of the Integrated Health System, as part of the actions of the Pink October, in partnership with the General Directorate and the Procuradoria Especial da Mulher (Women's Special Attorneyship). There were 150 openings, and they were quickly taken. Women aged 40 or over were selected for consults with doctors from the Senate and with Doctor Carlos Marino, from the Brazilian Society of Mastology, all assisted by the Regional Hospital of Asa Norte in order to investigate the possibility of breast cancer (**Figure 4**).

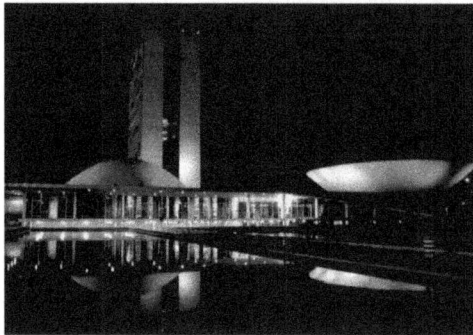

Figure 2. Special lighting of the National Congress (photo by Pillar Pedreira, Senado Federal).

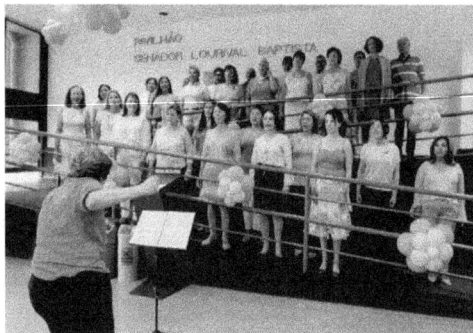

Figure 3. Choral presentation at the Pink October event (photo by Stumpf F, Senado Federal).

The hall of the Medical Service building was decorated with pink balloons to receive the collaborators. They were then invited for a nice breakfast, which was only made possible from the donations of the Senate's Civil Servants. They also counted on the support of the Occupational Health Service and the Quality of Life at Work department to do labor gymnastics. Late in the morning, the Senate Choir gave a presentation at the venue of the event (**Figure 3**).

The following events took place throughout the month of October (**Figure 5**):

- October Rosa against Breast Cancer—Ceremony of lighting of the National Congress.

- Artistic presentation of the Etude Seasons Ballet School with "Sleeping Beauty" by Tchaikovsky.

- Seminar to discuss the implementation of Law 12.732 / 2012, which determines a period of up to 60 days from the diagnosis for cancer patients to start treatment.

- "Talk Show" of the Oncovida Institute on Breast Cancer Prevention.

- Glamorous Parade from the "Roses of the Cerrado" (Victorious Women of Brasilia Against Breast Cancer)

- Consultation for outsourced women employees to undergo mammography at the Regional Hospital of Asa Norte.

- Women's Health Workshop: Autonomy in the Body and in Life

- Human Pink Tie for Life

- Performative act of parliamentarians and leaders for the prevention of breast cancer.

- Public Hearing: "Advances in coping with breast cancer in Brazil: health promotion, prevention, detection and availability of treatment."

- Women's Agenda: "II National Conference on Women's Health - Results and Challenges."

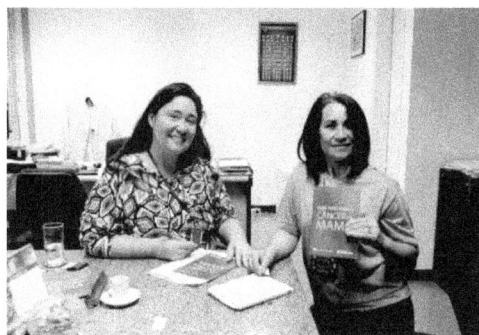

Figure 4. Toward a specific target (photo by Stumpf F, Senado Federal).

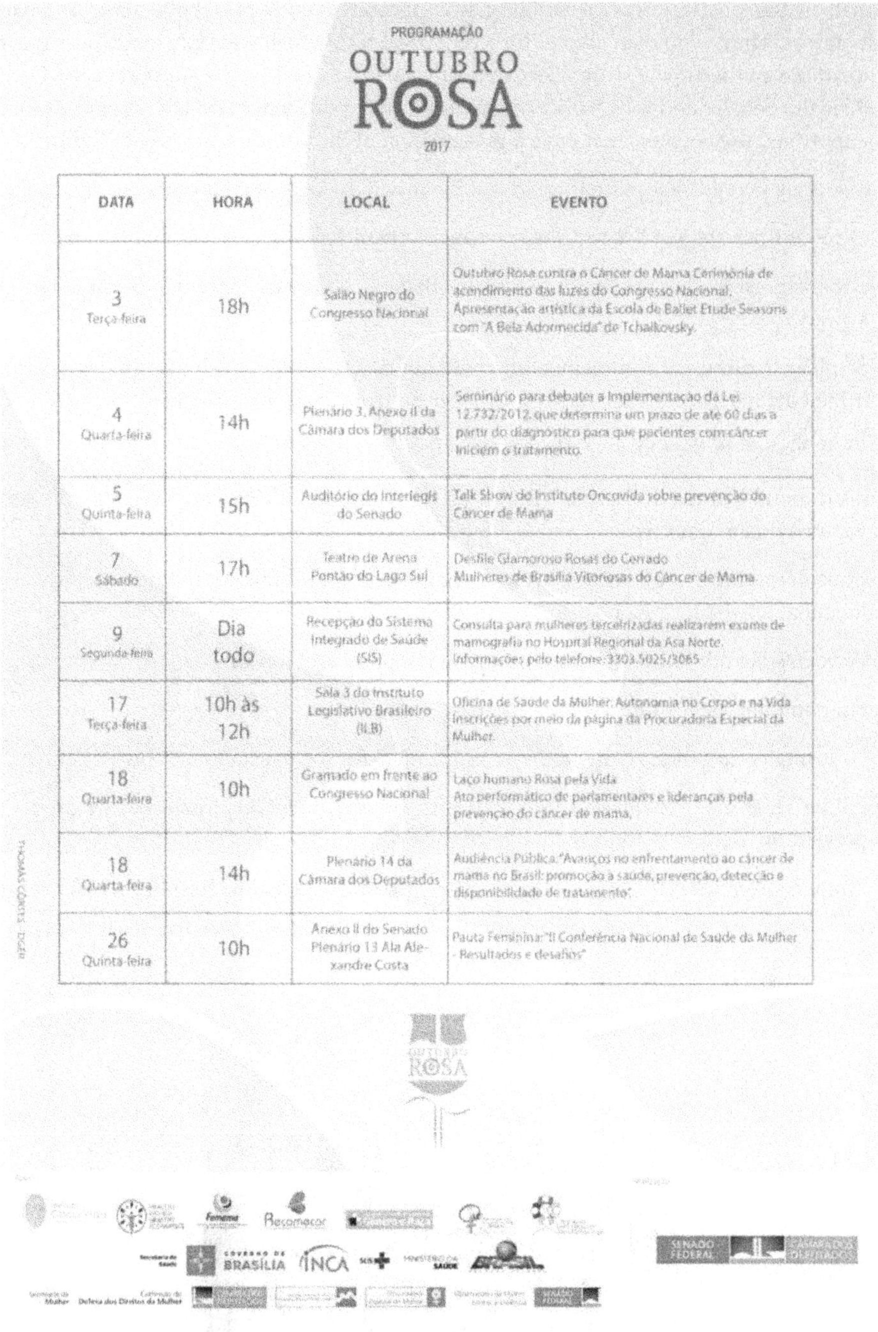

PROGRAMAÇÃO

OUTUBRO ROSA

2017

DATA	HORA	LOCAL	EVENTO
3 Terça-feira	18h	Salão Negro do Congresso Nacional	Outubro Rosa contra o Câncer de Mama Cerimônia de acendimento das luzes do Congresso Nacional. Apresentação artística da Escola de Ballet Etude Seasons com "A Bela Adormecida" de Tchaikovsky.
4 Quarta-feira	14h	Plenário 3, Anexo II da Câmara dos Deputados	Seminário para debater a Implementação da Lei 12.732/2012, que determina um prazo de até 60 dias a partir do diagnóstico para que pacientes com câncer iniciem o tratamento.
5 Quinta-feira	15h	Auditório do Interlegis do Senado	Talk Show do Instituto Oncovida sobre prevenção do Câncer de Mama
7 Sábado	17h	Teatro de Arena Pontão do Lago Sul	Desfile Glamoroso Rosas do Cerrado Mulheres de Brasília Vitoriosas do Câncer de Mama.
9 Segunda-feira	Dia todo	Recepção do Sistema Integrado de Saúde (SIS)	Consulta para mulheres tercerizadas realizarem exame de mamografia no Hospital Regional da Asa Norte. Informações pelo telefone: 3303.5025/3065
17 Terça-feira	10h às 12h	Sala 3 do Instituto Legislativo Brasileiro (ILB)	Oficina de Saúde da Mulher: Autonomia no Corpo e na Vida Inscrições por meio da página da Procuradoria Especial da Mulher.
18 Quarta-feira	10h	Gramado em frente ao Congresso Nacional	Laço humano Rosa pela Vida Ato performático de parlamentares e lideranças pela prevenção do câncer de mama.
18 Quarta-feira	14h	Plenário 14 da Câmara dos Deputados	Audiência Pública: "Avanços no enfrentamento ao câncer de mama no Brasil: promoção à saúde, prevenção, detecção e disponibilidade de tratamento".
26 Quinta-feira	10h	Anexo II do Senado Plenário 13 Ala Alexandre Costa	Pauta Feminina: "II Conferência Nacional de Saúde da Mulher - Resultados e desafios"

Figure 5. Pink October full program.

3.3. Media and assessment

In order to maximize the range and reach of the Pink October 2017 Program, the Federal Senate concatenated several complementary media, such as the Intranet, the Federal Senate's newspaper, television channel, radio station, web agency, Instagram, Facebook, Twitter and Tumblr, along with electronic mail and printed banners.

Two specific posts were published on the Senate's official Facebook page in October 2017 (**Figures 6** and **7**).

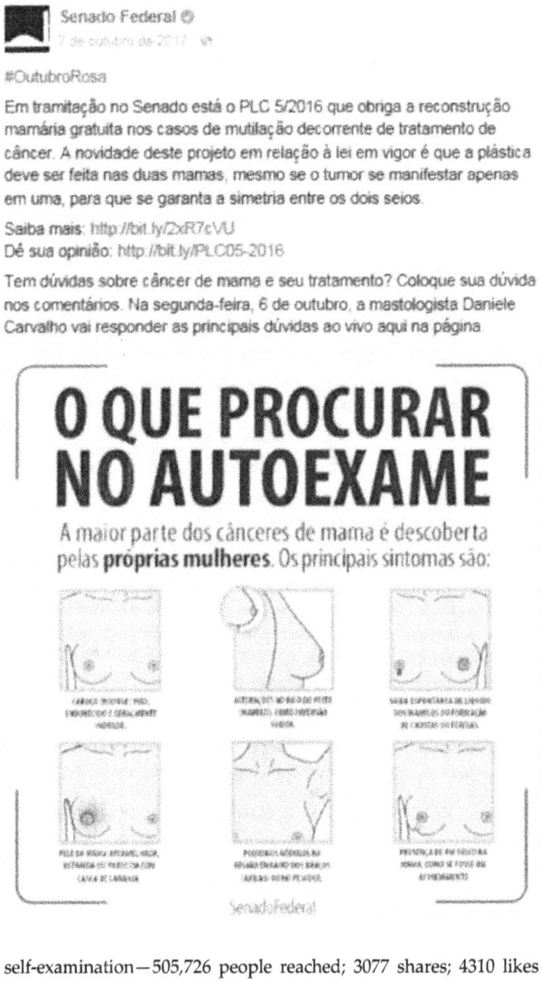

Senado Federal
7 de outubro de 2017

#OutubroRosa

Em tramitação no Senado está o PLC 5/2016 que obriga a reconstrução mamária gratuita nos casos de mutilação decorrente de tratamento de câncer. A novidade deste projeto em relação à lei em vigor é que a plástica deve ser feita nas duas mamas, mesmo se o tumor se manifestar apenas em uma, para que se garanta a simetria entre os dois seios.

Saiba mais: http://bit.ly/2xR7cVU
Dê sua opinião: http://bit.ly/PLC05-2016

Tem dúvidas sobre câncer de mama e seu tratamento? Coloque sua dúvida nos comentários. Na segunda-feira, 6 de outubro, a mastologista Daniele Carvalho vai responder as principais dúvidas ao vivo aqui na página

O QUE PROCURAR NO AUTOEXAME

A maior parte dos cânceres de mama é descoberta pelas **próprias mulheres**. Os principais sintomas são:

Figure 6. Tips on breast self-examination—505,726 people reached; 3077 shares; 4310 likes (Legend: Federal Senate/ October 7, 2017/ #OutubroRosa).

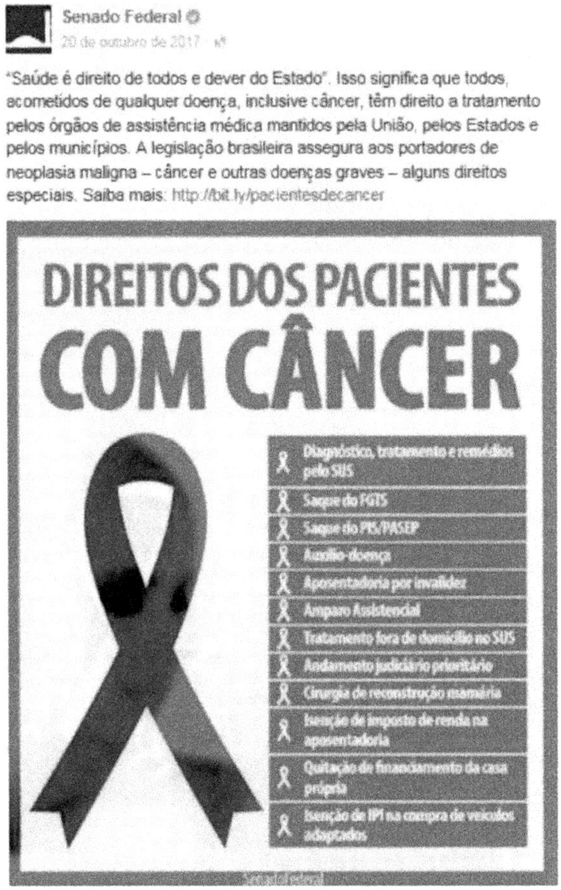

Senado Federal ☺
20 de outubro de 2017 · ✎

"Saúde é direito de todos e dever do Estado". Isso significa que todos, acometidos de qualquer doença, inclusive câncer, têm direito a tratamento pelos órgãos de assistência médica mantidos pela União, pelos Estados e pelos municípios. A legislação brasileira assegura aos portadores de neoplasia maligna – câncer e outras doenças graves – alguns direitos especiais. Saiba mais: http://bit.ly/pacientesdecancer

DIREITOS DOS PACIENTES
COM CÂNCER

- Diagnóstico, tratamento e remédios pelo SUS
- Saque do FGTS
- Saque do PIS/PASEP
- Auxílio-doença
- Aposentadoria por invalidez
- Amparo Assistencial
- Tratamento fora de domicílio no SUS
- Andamento judiciário prioritário
- Cirurgia de reconstrução mamária
- Isenção de imposto de renda na aposentadoria
- Quitação de financiamento da casa própria
- Isenção de IPI na compra de veículos adaptados

Figure 7. Rights of cancer patients—417,000 people reached; 3953 shares; 5016 likes. [Legend: "The right to health is a right for everybody and the duty of the state." This means that everyone affected by any disease, including cancer, is entitled to treatment by the health care agencies maintained by the Union, the States and the municipalities. Brazilian legislation ensures special rights to people who have malignant neoplasms, such as cancer and other serious diseases. Learn more: http://bit.ly/pacientesdecancer].

In the Senate, the bill 5/2016 which obliges the free breast reconstruction in cases of mutilation arising from cancer treatment is currently in progress. The innovation of this project in relation to the law in force is that the plastic surgery should be done on both breasts, even if the tumor manifests only in one, so that the symmetry between the two breasts is guaranteed.

Learn more: http://bit.ly/2xR7cVU /Give your opinion: http://bit.ly/PLC05-2016

Do you have any questions about breast cancer and its treatment? Type your question in the comments. On Monday, October 6th, the Mastologist Doctor Daniele Carvalho will answer the main questions live, here on the page.

What to look for in the self-exam?

Most breast cancers are discovered by women themselves.

The main symptoms are:

A nodule (lump), hardened and usually painless.

Changes in the appearance of the nipple, such as sudden nipple reversal.

Spontaneous discharge of nipple or formation of scabs or wounds.

Reddish breast skin. Retracted or similar to orange peel.

Small nodules in the region under the arms (armpits) or neck.

Inward dimpling of the breast tissue, as if there was an indentation).

In addition, Facebook and Twitter avatars (profile images) as well as the covers were temporarily changed.

The Senate also produced a series of videos on the importance of breast cancer prevention and control. In all, seven internal programs were presented by the mastologists Doctor Daniele Calvano and Doctor Martinho Cândido on topics such as heredity, risk factors and forms of treatment. The material was produced by TV Senado and by the General Coordination of Health, in connection with the Secretary of Human Resources.

The choice of the topics covered was based on the patients' main doubts, and the contents were defined by mastologists who work at the institution. The subjects that generate the most curiosity among the patients were then chosen.

In the doctors' point of view, knowledge is the first tool to prevent and fight the disease. If people know about the disease, they will not be afraid of the diagnosis, nor fear the treatment and are more likely to ask for help. In the case of breast cancer, early treatment guarantees a good chance of cure.

The Secretariat of Social Communication, responsible for the campaign videos, had the goal to offer citizens direct and attractive material. Therefore, the average duration of each inter-program was 30 s. The idea was to get a quick, informative message that could come in between TV shows.

The Procuradoria Especial da Mulher (Women's Special Attorneyship) also promoted initiatives both inside and outside the Federal Senate, supporting that its intention was to draw the population's attention to the fact that women must have access to the cancer diagnosis and treatment. Its main goal was to make everyone aware that the campaign had reached as many people as possible, through the use of social media.

The videos are available on YouTube and on the Senate portal.

https://www12.senado.leg.br/noticias/videos/2017/10/quais-os-fatores-de-risco-para-o-cancer--de-mama https://www.youtube.com/watch?v=BIHvRurHahE&list=PLLLnytnGoqiYLAs-jeepfk312REkzb1iE9

The link for the playlist page of Pink October on YouTube is

https://www.youtube.com/playlist?list=PLLLnytnGoqiYLAsjeepfk312REkzb1iE9

The seven videos on YouTube reached the following number of people:

1. How to prevent breast cancer = 391

2. Is all breast cancer hereditary? = 181

3. What are the genetic factors of breast cancer? = 101

4. What are the risk factors for breast cancer? = 337

5. Forms of treatment for breast cancer = 33

6. Breast reconstruction guaranteed by law = 27

7. How many new cancer cases occur in Brazil? = 23

A series of articles and news were published online on the Senate's Intranet. The titles and the reading access number are as follows:

- Outubro Rosa: vídeos produzidos pelo Senado auxiliam na prevenção ao câncer de mama (Pink October: Videos produced by the Senate help in preventing breast cancer): 19 views

- Outubro Rosa alerta para necessidade do diagnóstico precoce do câncer (Pink October alert to the need for early diagnosis of cancer): 781 views

- Outubro Rosa é aberto com alerta sobre importância da prevenção contra o câncer (Pink October opening with warning about the importance of cancer prevention): 418 views

- Terceirizadas passam por triagem no SIS para fazer mamografia gratuitamente (Outsourcers undergo triage in SIS for free mammography): 393 views

- Estilo de vida e herança genética podem causar câncer, afirmam especialistas (Lifestyle and genetic inheritance can cause cancer, experts say): 327 views

- Talk show com médicos, nesta quinta, discute a prevenção do câncer de mama (Talk show with doctors, this Thursday, discusses breast cancer prevention): 71 views

- Senado promove nesta quarta conversa pelo Facebook sobre câncer de mama (This coming Wednesday, the Senate promotes conversation by Facebook about breast cancer): 48 views

With a much broader target, the Senate's homepage on the Internet reached results as shown below for the following news:

Title	Type	Total access (through social media and search engines)
Outubro Rosa conscientiza sobre prevenção do câncer de mama (Pink October raises awareness on breast cancer prevention)	Special TV Show Cidadania. 10/03/2017	1738
Senado promove nesta terça conversa pelo Facebook sobre câncer de mama (This coming Thursday, the Senate promotes conversation by Facebook about breast cancer)	News Article 10/10/2017	272
Outubro Rosa visa desmistificar o câncer de mama, afirma médica (Pink October aims to demystify breast cancer, says doctor)	Video 10/13/2017	88
Como prevenir o câncer de mama? (How to prevent breast cancer?)	Video 10/04/2017	157
Todo câncer de mama é hereditário? (Is every breast cancer case hereditary?)	Video 10/09/2017	261
Quais os fatores de risco para o câncer de mama? (What are the risk factors for breast cancer?)	Video 10/16/2017	123
Aberta campanha Outubro Rosa no Congresso Nacional (Pink October Campaign is released in the National Congress)	News article 10/03/2017	500

Although the target audience of the campaign has been the outsourced employees of the Senate, in terms of information and clarification, the campaign has reached a much broader internal and external audience, as shown by the visualization metrics of the activities.

When examining the campaign from the point of view of the 7 Ps of social marketing, according to Fine, and quoted by Bates [43], we have answers for the following questions:

(a) Who is the **Producer**, the source of the promotional message?

The Senate as well as expert partners were the message producers.

(b) Who makes up the potential **Purchasers** that we must address, and what needs and desires do these people have?

An immediate audience, composed of the outsourced employees without access to resources for medical tests, a wider audience composed of all the internal audience (other female servers in the Senate), and the general public, reached by the message, which is all the women who are part of the audience outside the Senate, who were reached either by social media, or by more traditional communication vehicles such as the radio, TV and newspaper.

(c) What Products can be identified specifically to meet those needs?

Basically the detailed information about breast cancer and its prevention, and the clinical and hospital tests and doctors consultations carried out.

(d) What is the **Price** the consumers will sacrifice to acquire the product?

In short, the price is the time available for the allocation of cognitive resources to get in contact, assimilate and share information, and also to face the fight against the fear; the fear of submitting oneself to medical tests, and to be prepared to eventually receive bad news regarding one's health in case of a positive diagnosis.

(e) How can we communicate with our markets (**Promote**)?

Social media and other communication vehicles in the traditional media of the Federal Senate were used, as well as its internal information network, such as the Intranet, corporate emails and banners spread throughout the institution, in addition to events and artistic performances.

(f) Which institutions are involved in the process of making the product available at the best time and **Place**, for the buyer?

The internal infrastructure of the health service of the Federal Senate was provided, in partnership with the infrastructure of public health, at the time of the tests.

(g) How can we **Probe** and evaluate the campaign and how can feedback from the public be obtained?

Metrics for disclosure, visualization, and reviews of materials and postings were evaluated, as well as spontaneous manifestations of participants.

4. Conclusion

According to Mowen and Minor, research can benefit society. "Finding ways to influence people to act more responsibly [...] and applying research findings to develop treatment methods and preventive actions" is paramount, and the natural way to do this is through the research into social marketing best practices [42].

Considering the campaign analyzed in this chapter, besides the health communication informing about breast cancer, several other actions took place. A major effort was made in order to reach Brazilian citizens through the Senate's social media, as well as with an actual person-to-person contact, all these to try to make more people aware of the disease. For that, a close-targeted initiative was developed throughout the month of October: the outsourced female collaborators were invited to undergo an on-site medical consultation with the Senate mastologist doctors, and if the case required, the patient would be referred to a mammography exam carried out by the Public Health System (as a result of the partnership between the Senate and the Federal District Government). A total of 150 mammograms were performed. A disturbing fact is that most of the women who were reached by the initiative had never undergone a mammography before, which is an important exam to prevent breast cancer.

From the 150 patients assisted, 15 had an altered mammography result, and 4 of them had a diagnosis of breast cancer and were referred to a public hospital for treatment.

Although 150 people is a limited audience, the tests and the mammograms were just part of the campaign, which aimed to achieve, through advertising and journalistic information, the awareness of a wider audience, and the numbers registered show the campaign was extremely successful.

The high point of the initiative was being able to have the full support of the Public Health System to conduct the exams. It was a very important strategic partnership for the 2017 campaign, one that must be cherished and nurtured. Nevertheless, some mammograms were not performed within the expected period, due to problems commonly found in public hospitals nationwide, such as lack of personnel and equipment availability. This issue should be carefully addressed in the future editions of the Pink October campaign, for a more precise logistics and service for the women targeted in the program.

Other public and private institutions can take advantage of the strategies—and, literally, of all the informational materials produced –, although adjustments on the brand are needed, specially due to the fact that the October Rosa brand in the Senate has used the silhouette of the building of the National Congress.

Acknowledgements

The authors would like to thank Mr. Mikhail Lopes and Mr. Eduardo Leão, from the Secretariat of Social Communication of the Federal Senate, for their valuable assistance in gathering metrics from the Senate's social media and from Intranet news, and of the Certified Translator Elisângela Tarouco for the context and grammar review.

Author details

Paulo Ricardo dos Santos Meira[1,2,3*], Ilana Trombka[2,3,4] and
Daniele Carvalho Calvano Mendes[2]

*Address all correspondence to: paulomeira@gmail.com

1 Universidade Federal do Rio Grande do Sul, Brazil

2 Brazilian Federal Senate, Brazil,

3 Instituto Legislativo Brasileiro (ILB), Brazil

4 Board Council of the Senate's Health Integrated System, Brazil

References

[1] Sheth J, Frazier G. A model of strategy mix for planned social change. Journal of Marketing. 1982;**46**(1, Winter):15-26

[2] Andreasen A. The life trajectory of social marketing: Some implications. Marketing Theory [SAGE]. 2003, 2003;**3**:293-303. DOI: 10.1177/147059310333004

[3]   Davis KC, Evans WD, Kamyab K. Effectiveness of a national media campaign to promote parent-child communication about sex. Health Education and Behavior. 2013;**40**(1):97-106. DOI: 10.1177/1090198112440009

[4]   Kotler P, Roberto N, Lee N. Social Marketing: Improving the Quality of Life. 2nd. ed. CA: Sage Publications; 2002. ISBN-10: 0761924345

[5]   Outubro Rosa conscientiza sobre prevenção do câncer de mama [Internet]. Interview with Dr. Daniele Carvalho Calvano Mendes. 2017. Available from: http://www.seceto.com.br/outubro-rosa-conscientiza-sobre-prevencao-do-cancer-de-mama/ [Accessed: 2018-01-07]

[6]   Shimp TA. Advertising, Promotion and Other Aspects of Integrated Marketing Communications, 8th ed. Cengage Learning; 2008

[7]   Meira PRS, Santos CP. Social marketing programs in Brazil: Metrics and social media approaches. In: Evans WD, org. Social Marketing: Global Perspectives, Strategies and Effects on Consumer Behavior, v. 1. 1st ed. New York: Nova Science Publishers; 2017. pp. 147-178. ISBN: 978-1-63485-780-2

[8]   Kotler P, Lee N. Marketing in the 7Public Sector: a Roadmap for Improved Performance. Pearson Education; 2007. ISBN-13: 9780137060863

[9]   Wilkie W, Moore E. Scholarly research in marketing: Exploring the "4 eras" of thought development. Journal of Public Policy & Marketing. 2003;**22**(2):116-146. DOI: 10.1509/jppm.22.2.116.17639

[10] Ling JC, Franklin BAK, Lindsteadt JF, Gearon SAN. Social marketing: Its place in public health. Annual Review of Public Health. May 1992;**13**:341-362

[11] Gordon R, McDermott L, Stead M, Angus K. The effectiveness of social marketing interventions for health improvement: What's the evidence? Public Health. 2006;**120**(12):1133-1139. DOI: 10.1016/j.puhe.2006.10.008

[12] Andreasen A. Ethics in Social Marketing. Georgetown University Press; 2001. 212 p. ISBN: 0878408207

[13] Cooksy LJ. Evaluators' Reflections on the Ethical Implications of Their Early Experiences. American Journal of Evaluation. Sage Publications; 2009. DOI: 10.1177/1098214009349794

[14] Brenkert G. Ethical challenges of social marketing. Journal of Public Policy & Marketing. 2002;**21**(1):14–25. DOI: 10.1509/jppm.21.1.14.17601

[15] Kotler P, Lee N. Marketing no Setor Público: um guia para um desempenho mais eficaz. Porto Alegre: Bookman; 2008. 350 p

[16] Bates C. Use of social marketing concepts to evaluate ocean sustainability campaigns. Social Marketing Quarterly. 2010;**16**(1):71-96

[17] Peters DH, Mirchandani GG, Hansen P. Strategies for engaging the private sector in sexual and reproductive health: How effective are they? Health Policy and Planning. 2004;**19**:I5

[18] Haider M. Global Public Health Communications: Challenges, Perspectives, and Strategies. Sudbury, MA: Jones & Bartlett Publishers; 2005

[19] Hastings G. Relational paradigms in social marketing. Journal of Macromarketing. 2003; **23**(1):6-15

[20] Bozzetti N. Brands and Internal Communication. [Speech] at Centro Universitário Ritter dos Reis. Porto Alegre, Brazil; 2003

[21] Evans WD, Hastings G, editors. Public Health Branding: Applying Marketing for Social Change. Oxford: Oxford University Press; 2008. ISBN: 978-0-19-923713-5

[22] Keller KL. Branding perspectives on social marketing. Advances in Consumer Research. Vol. 25. In: Alba JW, Wesley Hutchinson J, editors. Provo, UT: Association for Consumer Research; 1998. pp. 299-302

[23] Evans WD, editor. Psychology of Branding. Nova Science Publishers: NY; 2013

[24] Gronroos C. Service, Management and Marketing. Toronto DC Health and Company: Lexington, MA; 1990

[25] Kotler P, Keller KL. Marketing Management. 14th ed. New Jersey, USA: Prentice Hall; 2012

[26] Costa D. Relatório Brasil de Endomarketing e Comunicação Interna. Porto Alegre: Santo de Casa Endomarketing. Edição 2012/2013; 2013. 76 p

[27] Kerin RA, Hartley SW, Berkowitz EN, Rudelius W. Marketing. 8th ed. New York, USA: McGraw-Hill Irwin; 2006

[28] Carvajal L. Fundamentos de la Imagen Visual Corporativa. E-book. Astrolabio; 2013. Available from: https://itunes.apple.com/br/book/fundamentos-la-imagen-visual/id547151324?mt=11 [Accessed: 2018-02-10]

[29] Dias L. O Desafio no Setor Público. In: Costa D, org. Relatório Brasil de Endomarketing e Comunicação Interna. Porto Alegre: Santo de Casa Endomarketing. Edição 2012/2013; 2013. pp. 72-76

[30] Evans WD, Holtz K, Snider J. Effects of the above the influence brand on adolescent drug use prevention beliefs. Journal of Health Communication. 2014;**19**(6):721-737. DOI: 10.1080/10810730.2013.837559

[31] Valente J. Relatório aponta Brasil como quarto país em número de usuários de internet. Agência Brasil. Oct. 10, 2017. Available from: http://agenciabrasil.ebc.com.br/geral/noticia/ 2017-10/relatorio-aponta-brasil-como-quarto-pais-em-numero-de-usuarios-de-internet [Accessed: 2018-02-01]

[32] Brasil é o maior usuário de redes sociais da América Latina. Revista Forbes. June 20, 2016. Available from: http://forbes.uol.com.br/fotos/2016/06/brasil-e-o-maior-usuario-de-redes-sociais-da-america-latina/ [Accessed: 2018-02-01]

[33] Jornal do Senado. Seminário mostra como redes sociais na internet têm interferido na política. Brasília; 2012, 9 July. Cover and p. 2

[34] Williamson A. Social Media Guidelines for Parliaments. 2013. Available from: http://www.andywilliamson.com/index.php/social-media-guidelines-for-parliaments/ [Accessed: 2018-01-25]

[35] Senado Federal. Modernidade no Senado Federal: Presidências de José Sarney. Brasília: Senado Federal. 2012. 270 p. Available from: http://www.senado.gov.br/senado/modernidade/pdf/Modernidade_digital.pdf. [Accessed: 2018-01-10]

[36] Cidadão poderá se comunicar com o Senado por meio das redes sociais. Jornal do Senado. 2011;**IX**(334):Especial Cidadania, 1° Febr

[37] Senado Federal. Portfólio de Trabalhos Institucionais 2009–2013 da Coordenação de Publicidade e Marketing. Brasília: Senado Federal; 2013

[38] Schellong A. Citizen Relationship Management. In: Anttiroiko A, Malkia M, editors. Encyclopedia of Digital Government. London: Idea Group Inc.; 2007. Available from: http://www.hks.harvard.edu/netgov/files/alex/schellong_2007_edog_article_citizen_relationship_management_311_call_center_egovernment.pdf [Accessed: 2018-01-05]

[39] Redes sociais ampliam alcance de público das informações produzidas pelo Senado. Intranet Senado Federal. April 26, 2017. Available from: https://intranet.senado.leg.br/noticias/materias/2016/06/redes-sociais-ampliam [Accessed: 2018-02-02]

[40] Trombka I. Carta de Gestão dos 33 Meses. [Internal e-mail communication at the Federal Senate as a management report]. Brasília: Senado Federal; 10 Nov, 2017

[41] Outubro Rosa conscientiza sobre prevenção do câncer de mama. November 7, 2017. Available from: http://www.seceto.com.br/outubro-rosa-conscientiza-sobre-prevencao-do-cancer-de-mama/. [Accessed: 2018-02-15]

[42] Mowen J, Minor M. Consumer Behavior: A Framework. New Jersey, USA: Prentice Hall; 2000

[43] Bates D. Book Review on Social Marketing: Strategies for Changing Public Behavior by Philip Kotler and Eduardo L. Roberto, and Social Marketing: Promoting the Causes of Public and Nonprofit Agencies by Fine SH. Journal of Marketing. January 1991